# Adult Autism

# Adult Autism

*A journey, and
some thoughts*

JON VENFORD-BROWN

VB Books

First published 2018 by VB Books 2018



Typeset 11pt Lucida Bright

ISBN-13: 978-1720857051
ISBN-10: 1720857059

Cover design based on *Anxiety*, Edvard Munch

Printed by CreateSpace

# Contents

# Contents

# Introduction

It seems that only a few years ago I was completely unaware of the terms autism and Asperger syndrome. I had however realised that some people I met were slightly 'different' – on the face of it, possibly a rather superficial or even crass comment, as we are all different. As my wife puts it rather more articulately, certain people are 'not wired quite the same'.

Although I suppose I had long had some indefinable feeling at the back of my mind that something I could not put my finger on was not quite right, I was one of them. At length, as related below, I was diagnosed myself in my late fifties. Better late than never.

An old friend from my student days, a librarian (now retired) by profession who has also worked as a bereavement visitor and counsellor, says that there are many people on the edge of the autism spectrum. It is a broad one ranging from very severe to very mild, and there is no hard and fast dividing line between people who are on it and those who are neurotypical (neurologically typical), allistic, or in plain old-fashioned terms, 'normal'. For a long time, the literature on it was sparse because of what might be called a 'wall of silence' on mental health conditions and what is actually a mental health issue.

This situation has changed in recent years, but nevertheless I felt there was a shortage of books about autism from the adult point of view. Having worked in a college of further and higher education for some years, it was evident that most of what was available was focused on the condition as regards children, and on helping parents to deal with it. A colleague with whom I discussed the matter fully agreed with me. As children tend to be diagnosed around the time they start school, this is not surprising. As I read more thoroughly into the subject and trawled the online sources available, it became clear that many adults were realising they were similarly affected, had unknowingly struggled for some years with an inner sense that something was not quite right, and in some cases only found out because they shared the same difficulties as their child who had just received a diagnosis.

In 2015, it was reported that an increased awareness about autism was behind a boom in diagnosis rates, estimated to affect more than one in 100 people in the United Kingdom. Males were four times as likely to be diagnosed as women, who might be on the spectrum but were considered more adept at copying social norms. 'Girls are definitely better at hiding it,' according to Hannah Khan, speaking during her first year at university. 'They might get missed. A lot of people who don't get diagnosed, almost don't want to be diagnosed. They don't want a diagnosis because it's a bad thing. But it's a step towards getting help.'[1] Other young women, often in their twenties, have initially been told by their doctor that they have BPO (borderline personality disorder), and all they need is a quick fix – 'here's the prescription, just take the tablets'. Only their gut feeling has led them to persevere for a proper diagnosis.

It is sometimes accepted that nearly all of us have one or two mildly autistic traits. Some of us have several, while others have so many that they may find it difficult to function normally. Such people would have been unfairly castigated as idiots in a time before autism was fully recognised. There are many shades in between. Until not so long ago it was hard, if not impossible, for adults to get a diagnosis even in the worst cases. Higher functioning ones were merely seen as eccentric, and no help was available. Initially it was blamed on poor mothering, perhaps as a number of mothers of severely autistic children were mildly affected themselves.

For people in their thirties and upwards who were recognising the autistic traits of their small sons and daughters in themselves, according to Carol Povey, director of the National Autistic Centre's Centre for Autism, it could be a milestone in their life. 'It provides an explanation for feeling 'different' after years of not understanding why they found some things difficult or thought differently from their peers. It's also a gateway to identifying essential support.' She also believes that in the past it was seen as a childhood condition, a perception which still persists. Many adults, she says, have 'been diagnosed with depression, anxiety, borderline personality disorders and drug or alcohol issues without recognition that autism lay at the root of their problems.'[2]

My progression towards the light at the end of the tunnel, to coin a phrase, was different. I never had children, and to be honest I never wanted to be a parent. As I sometimes told others, I did not marry at haste and repent at leisure, my bachelor life having come to an end in my late forties. It was my wife who, bless her, realised a few months into our togetherness that there were issues to be addressed.

Several years on, I hope that my experience, and what at the risk of sounding slightly pretentious is an ongoing journey of self-discovery, will prove of interest and even help to others. My conversations with a few close friends, some of whom had a keen interest and practical hands-on experience of the subject, although not autistic themselves, convinced me that there was a need for this book. Maybe someone reading this will find that they are ticking a number of the boxes themselves, or on behalf of a friend or member of the family. In that case, I will feel that this has achieved something positive.

I am not by any stretch of the imagination what might be termed a 'health professional', and have never formally studied health, psychology or anything of the kind. Such knowledge as I have acquired has come through reading, talking to and exchanging views with others who are usually much better-informed than I am, and surfing the net. Since I began writing this, I have learnt a good deal in a very short time. So do not expect a plethora of specialised scientific terms or jargon. Other books on the subject will cater for that need, if need it is, far better than this book will.

Talking of which, the available literature on autism and Asperger syndrome is vast, and growing all the time. It would be easy for me to feel guilty when somebody asks 'have you read so-and-so's book', and I have to shake my head, wondering if I should admit to having never even heard of it. There is likewise enough material online, if not more than enough. I have purposely restricted myself to a select handful of resources, as much for background reading and amplification of the basic facts as anything else. These are cited as necessary in the references.

As developments regarding strategies for diagnosis, treatment and everything else relating to the subject are constantly evolving, I felt there was little to be gained in reproducing wholesale vast amounts of information which may be out of date by the time it is in print, or very soon afterwards. There is no substitute for seeking out up-to-date details online. Nevertheless, I hope that a book such as this will find a place on the bookshelves of those who wish to know more.

# What are Autism, Asperger syndrome, and what is the difference?

Autism is not a single condition, but rather a spectrum of disorders that affects people in various ways and to different degrees. As it is a set of conditions and not a physical disability, there is no medical test that will reveal whether somebody is autistic or not. It is not a mental illness, although there has long been a stigma attached to mental disability in all its forms, and is perhaps close enough to it for some people to think of autistic people differently – and perhaps negatively. Autistic spectrum conditions are lifelong neurodevelopmental disorders, and a diagnosis is based on the presence of multiple symptoms. Characteristics of those who are on the autism spectrum include a love of routines, difficulty with social interaction, special interests, repetitive behaviours and sensory problems such as with noise or textures. Sometimes defined as the 'triad of impairments', these comprise:

- Social interactions, or problems understanding the perspectives and emotions of others. Autistic people find

it difficult to interact with and talk to
other people socially, or perhaps talking
at length about their special interests
without allowing others the chance to
join in, being seemingly oblivious to
knowledge of appropriate behaviour in
particular circumstances, and unable to
form friendships with ease. Sometimes
they can recognise and overcome this to
an extent by developing a friendly
manner, but not without the effort which
may involve masking a feeling of internal
panic

- Verbal and non-verbal communication
  difficulties. People have problems in
  understanding and interpreting the
  feelings of others, because of a blind spot
  as regards facial expression, body
  language or tone of voice and thus
  misreading their mood. They tend to rely
  on very precise written instructions such
  as cheat-sheets, when attempting tasks
  with which they are unfamiliar, such as
  carrying out basic everyday procedures
  on a computer at work, or a washing
  machine at home

- Repetitive behaviour, such as repeating
  certain words or behaviours in a rigid
  rule-governed manner, or stimming, the
  repetition of physical movements,
  sounds, or repetitive movement of
  objects for no apparent purpose. People
  may not engage in games or activities
  that involve the use of imagination,
  preferring repetitive activities, or else
  copy the imaginative activities of others,

but without any genuine understanding.
They may have a love of routines, doing
certain things a particular way all the
time, and feeling more comfortable as a
result

Such definitions are not watertight. Most people on the spectrum will share some if not necessarily all of these, and not always to the same degree, but they often go together to a certain extent. One major misconception is that autistic people are generally supposed to lack empathy. This is not strictly true; what they usually lack is the ability to show and communicate it effectively, or fail to respond appropriately – a very different matter altogether. Sometimes people inadvertently give the wrong impression by shutting themselves off emotionally as a defence mechanism, in order to avoid getting hurt. Adults who are on the spectrum are sometimes perceived by others as having the emotional maturity of a teenager. They can become irritable over comparatively trivial matters, but often remain calm in a crisis when others panic.

An estimated ten per cent of individuals on the spectrum, many of these being of average or above average intelligence, demonstrate savant talents. These include such abilities as being able to count exceptionally fast, or carry out swift calculations as to the day of a week on which someone was born if told that person's date of birth.

People with autism have a brain that is developed differently, they see the world in a different way from others, and thus may have difficulty in communicating and forming relationships with others.[3] One definition uses the metaphor of the typical brain being like a fast road network, with information coming in at A going to B by travelling along the neural pathways, and like a car travelling along the motorways, the information gets to its destination without any problem. The autistic brain is different in that information coming in at A goes to B, but takes longer because of the differences in the brain like a car going from A to B along B roads, perhaps even getting lost and ending up at the seaside, C, turning up at its original destination weeks or even months later.[4]

As for Asperger syndrome, according to Dr Valerie Gaus, a practising cognitive-behavioural therapist, this is not a disease or a defect, but a set of differences.[5] While I was on my own road to diagnosis, or voyage of discovery, the two professionals who started the process said there were grounds for believing I had Asperger syndrome. The two who completed the task more than a year later concluded it was autism.

So what exactly is the difference? In general, Asperger syndrome tends to be regarded as the form not associated with learning difficulties, although it is less clear-cut than that. Let me paraphrase from a post I found on The Exclusive Inclusive Employment Hub blog, which tells us that people in whom Asperger's is identified at a young age do not experience delayed language development. This is considered to be a key difference between autism or autism spectrum disorder (ASD) and Asperger syndrome (AS). Moreover, people with Asperger's can function fairly well in everyday life, but tend to be socially immature, may be perceived by those around them as odd or eccentric, and tend to have an obsession with random things. Those with autism, or pervasive developmental disorders (PDD), generally suffer from five disorders characterized by varying degrees of impairment in communication skills and social interactions, as well as restricted, repetitive and stereotyped behaviours, and tend to have stronger connections with certain things, but not on the level of obsession. People with Asperger's may struggle with communication, but can be and often are brilliant at certain things.[6]

Another source gives us a more succinct pair of dictionary definitions. Autism is 'a mental condition characterised by great difficulty in communicating with others and in using language and abstract concepts', while Asperger syndrome is 'a mild autistic disorder characterised by awkwardness in social interaction, pedantry in speech, and preoccupation with very narrow interests'.[7]

A third source suggests that low-functioning autism relates to those who are less able, and is more or less synonymous with a lower than average IQ. Such people are said to show Kanner syndrome or 'classic autism' as they fit the description of children studied by Dr Leo Kanner [see below, p. 82-3]. High-functioning people, who are more able and have a higher than average IQ, display symptoms similar to those described by Hans Asperger [see below, p. 83-4]. While they may still have difficulties with language and communication, these are not nearly as marked as those shown by people at the low end of the spectrum. They generally have an extremely good command of language and a very rich vocabulary.

The post-diagnostic information pack with which I was supplied after my official diagnosis states succinctly that the diagnosis of Asperger syndrome is given to people who show the main features of the autism spectrum, but who do not have a history of delayed development, and have average or above average intelligence. It also mentions that 'you will hear some people refer to Asperger syndrome or High Functioning Autism as "mild forms of autism"', which is incorrect, as 'all people on the autism spectrum vary in terms of how they are affected by the symptoms of autism'.[8]

So how many different variations are there? Turning to a fifth – and this, I promise, will be the last before the old cliché 'let's not go there' floats somewhere across the horizon - the authors tell us some would contest that Asperger's and high functioning autism are different disorders, but for the purposes of their book both will be considered as part of the broader autism spectrum.[9]

Let us proceed with that. The more I have read myself while exploring the subject prior to my own referrals and diagnosis, and then later while writing this book, the more it seemed to me that there was a very fine line between the two. Savants may strongly disagree, but bearing in mind that the whole concept is relatively new and that the world has only gradually been waking up to the concepts and conditions of ASD and AS, I have found it hard not to consider the two as barely indistinguishable, and consider them more or less as one and the same throughout the book that follows.

Finally, autism diagnosis is not as precise as a diagnosis for some severe disease, but a behavioural profile. On the publication of the DSM-5, *The Diagnostic and Statistical Manual of Mental Disorders*, 5th edition), the 2013 update to the APAs (American Psychiatric Association) classification and diagnostic tool, the Asperger diagnosis was dropped as a distinct classification and merged into ASD. A new diagnosis was added, Social Communication Disorder, or Autism but without the repetitive behaviour or fixated interests.

Several studies over the last fifteen years or so have investigated the similarities and differences between the two disorders, using results from previous research. They compared various characteristics including language and communication, cognitive and neuropsychological profiles, motor skills, social behaviours and interests. The findings established that although there were differences in key behaviours, developmental course and symptoms to make them separate diagnoses, there was enough evidence to suggest an absence of differences. Despite these differences, there was enough evidence to encourage the idea that high-functioning autism and AS should be put under the same diagnosis. Both disorders are now under the same name, although there are still notable differences between the two. For example, people with Asperger's are as a rule more likely to go into details about emotions linked with problems relating to their difficulties, such as those connected with socialising with other people.[10]

It can be all too easy to pay excessive attention to these different classifications. Let us conclude with allowing Temple Grandin to have the last word. 'Do not get hung up on labels. Over the years, the doctors keep revising and changing the labels and their meaning .... Autism spectrum is a broad spectrum that ranges from very severe to merging into a personality variant at the far end of normal.'[11]

# My experience

How many times can you recall a friend saying to you as they look back on their childhood, maybe tongue in cheek, 'I was a strange child'? I probably have just as good reason as any. My earliest recollection, of which my memories are understandably vague, are of falling out of a window at the age of three, hitting my head and being rushed to hospital. I did not sustain any long-term physical injuries, although I assume there must have been the odd bruise or two, and as far as I know I was unharmed by the experience.

My mother used to tell me that I hardly spoke at all until I was about four. Whether they were seriously concerned at the time, or whether they thought I was a bit of a self-elective mute or not, is not mine to reason why. I was a passionate reader of books from about the same age, and had my head in one nearly all the time – something which has never changed very much, several decades later – and she also said that almost as soon as I started to speak, it was in full sentences. A few years later, again according to her, I had a habit of coming out with rather unusual words, as if – to use her phrase - I had swallowed a dictionary.

I enjoyed having my own space to what others might consider an extraordinary degree. One thing I was never allowed to live down was a birthday when I must have been about six or seven, and I took myself away from the scene of the party. After my guests had been entertained by my parents and elder sisters, I was discovered, quite unconcerned, having been curled up on my own - just reading. Maybe I had been given a particularly engrossing book that morning as a present, but it was probably by no means an isolated incident. I have vague memories of, when I was small, sometimes being quite annoyed when we were told we were to be taken out somewhere, or when people were coming to visit us and we had to be sociable. All I wanted was a quiet solitary time with my books, or maybe my stamps and coins. If not engaged in one of those activities, I was writing - short stories, poems, histories, even trying my hand at the occasional short play. If you gave me a pencil and a good supply of paper, you could leave me alone all day. I also had a love of setting general knowledge quizzes for the family, something which came in useful many years later when taking my turn in producing general and music questions at the local pub.

That leads me on to another subject. I also had my fair share, or perhaps more than that, of childhood obsessions, soaking up sometimes useless facts without any problem at all. Although I had forgotten about it by the time I was an adult, my parents told me that when I was little I had this bizarre facility of being able to work out in a few seconds what day of the week somebody was born on if they told me their date of birth – something which, perhaps fortunately, I completely lost a few years later. A family friend once told my parents that with this particular 'gift' I ought to have been on television. (Good grief, I could have been a child star ...) I can also remember being able to mop up historical dates like a sponge without trying. Ever since I was about five, I have been able to rattle off the dates of Kings and Queens since the Norman Conquest in my sleep. When I followed the family traditions of collecting stamps and coins, I acquired an almost encyclopaedic memory for the dates of specific issues. A few years later, when my lifelong love of pop and rock music began, it was chart positions of favourite groups and all their singles, even occasionally though not always specific catalogue numbers of particular releases, or the No 1 hits from a particular year in order. Collecting the catalogue numbers of early Penguin paperbacks, even to the extent of seeking them out in market stalls and large secondhand bookshops, became another of my peculiar passions when I was about twelve years old. A handful of them stick in my mind to this day. Fifty-something years later, I could have saved myself the trouble by going online and googling the whole lot. Sigh.

I suppose I have always had obsessive compulsive disorder in some ways. For example, at various times throughout my life, I have subconsciously counted and memorised the number of steps on various staircases in houses where I have lived or regularly stayed, or places where I have worked, and have been able to remember exactly how many there were a long time afterwards. Another point, connected with the love of and comfort in routines, is that I have often felt a little stressed or disoriented by sudden changes of plan, sometimes but not always during childhood, but more so as I have become older. I like to organise things in advance as far as possible, and find sudden alterations slightly disturbing, even disorientating. Living with other people who thrive on spontaneity inevitably entails some give and take and I can control this to a certain extent, but it does not come naturally.

This is all a little sad, I hear you say. Perhaps the saddest thing was that at one of my boarding schools, at the beginning of every term we were issued with a 'School Roll' in which everybody's name was printed, and alongside it their date of birth. Seemingly without trying, in my first or second term, I managed to memorise all these dates. Somehow the word got around, and in no time it was a case of 'Go and ask [me] when you were born.' (Did they not know themselves ... ) Of course, several of the staff got to hear about it. I wonder if they ever thought I was some kind of a freak, or to put it in more measured terms, not quite right. Forty or fifty years later, by which time everybody in education was aware of the spectrum, concerns might have been raised. I recall a school report produced by the headmistress of the primary school which I left when I was eight. It has long since been lost, but I remember her saying that I had marked interests in and was particularly knowledgeable about subjects such as history. Whether she had put her finger on any obsessive characteristics, I do not know. This was in 1962, when the theories of Hans Asperger and others were probably known only to a select few.

As I regularly came bottom of the form through being utterly hopeless at Mathematics and all science subjects, and was equally useless at games and sports at a school when sporting prowess was almost some kind of religion, there were times when I felt I did not have a lot going for me. Perhaps the extraordinary facility for absorbing mind-numbingly useless information proved something. I used to get bullied at school, long before Childline and so on, and did not cope with it very well. Those were the days when you had to take it on the chin and were left to cope with everything as best you could. More than anything else, I think my salvation was learning to play the guitar and writing songs. Nevertheless it did not save me from paranoia, or a constant feeling that I was being picked on, or criticised, disparaged, and found fault with behind my back.

At the age of fifteen, while I was revising for and sitting my O-level examinations, a combination of overwork and general miseries – perhaps my first real experience of reactive depression – resulted in some kind of a breakdown and even temporary alopecia or partial hair loss, although fortunately it did grow back within a few months. Only many years later, through my wife, did I learn that my mother had wanted to take me away from that school and find me another, but my father put my foot down and insisted I was staying put. I might have thought differently at the time, but in retrospect I know he made the right decision – and not just because in my final year, while preparing for A-levels, one term I wrote and acted in a one-act play, and also formed my first rock group who put on a gig in the school hall. Our peers loved it (I think), but I gathered it did not go down with the headmaster who frantically tried in vain to have the volume turned down – or off altogether. Very rock'n'roll. (On the other hand, as far as I know, he approved of the play). I did pass my A-levels, although not with the dazzlingly good grades that we all hoped might have been within my reach.

Something else I gradually learnt the hard way at school was to develop a sense of humour, become less earnest and not take everything literally or everyone too seriously. It became easier with experience, but I had the kind of personality to which it did not come naturally. Having said that, it is recognised that one of the characteristics of autism is humourlessness. Having discovered the books of P.G. Wodehouse and the films of Laurel and Hardy when I was about ten and adored them ever since, that is one box on the spectrum list I cannot tick.

From my teens onwards, for several years, I think I was relatively ordinary – well, most of the time. I spent two years at technical college in London, about two hundred miles from home, and lived in the hall of residence during termtime. One thing which slightly went over my head at the time it happened was when my mother was giving me and my luggage (if my English teachers are reading, sorry, my luggage and I) a lift to the station to put me on the Devon-London train for the first time. She told me that I would probably find the experience 'hellish', and that I must give it, say three weeks, and let her and my father know if I genuinely could not cope. Having spent the previous two years at home after the best part of ten years at two different boarding schools, I had no qualms about spending the next two years, punctuated by brief holidays at home, in the smoke. Only many years later did I wonder whether she had her suspicions about 'something'.

If so, she need not have lost any sleep over it. On balance I really enjoyed my time at college. I was very shy at first, and will never forget going to the first freshers' party a few days into the first term where I only knew one person, had a brief chat with him, then went and sat quietly in the corner partaking of the complimentary, seemingly unlimited liquid refreshment in a disposable plastic beaker. Only after several refills did I realise that it was a deceptively potent red wine. Somehow I staggered back afterwards to the hall of residence twenty minutes' walk away, hit the bed, and came to my senses about twelve hours later. And no, I did not take the pledge next day.

There were however times when I felt I needed to remove myself altogether from the company of others, and on most Saturdays I would take myself off to the centre of London to spend several hours on my own in art galleries, bookshops, record shops and general sites of interest. Looking back, I wonder if it was a form of social anxiety, long before any of us had ever heard of the term. In spite of that I made some very close and much-valued friends, most of them from the same lecture group as myself. Some of them were very different in personality from me, but we gelled together as a group extraordinarily well. Over forty years later, a few of us were/are still exchanging Christmas cards and short newsy letters.

I do remember one slight quirk I had which was commented on by somebody else, which I thought nothing of at the time but now seems to be part of a pattern. When I was arranging to meet a particular two or three friends the next day, I would say, 'see you at about such and such a time'. One of them noticed with increasing amusement that every time I did this, I would be bang on the time I had said I would - not a minute out either way. Eventually it got to the stage where I turned up one evening as punctual as ever and he roared with laughter. 'Bloody hell, Jon,' he said. 'Why do you ALWAYS have to be exactly on time?' Not long afterwards, I promised to ring him at his flat at about nine the following morning. Right on the dot, next day I picked up the phone in the Students' Union office and dialled him. This was long before the days of caller display on landlines – let alone mobile phones. A voice answered sleepily and greeted me by name. 'How did you know it was me?' I asked. 'It had to be – you're always on time,' was the reply.

Despite sort of falling in love with two different female students on my course who were happy to be pals but no more, I was sorry to leave the place at the end of my last term. Again, in the best student tradition rather a lot of alcohol went down the hatch on the final evening. Before I forget, thanks to the guys who saw me back to the hall of residence afterwards. I might not have managed it that easily without them.

Fast forward through a couple of short-lived relationships, which convinced my family that I was going to be a lifelong bachelor. After a brief spell of unemployment I worked successively in public and polytechnic (later university) libraries, the Land Registry, and then for many years in a college library. During that time I played and sang with rock groups on an amateur basis, worked on and off as a disc jockey, contributed articles and reviews to newspapers and magazines, and published several books, the majority being non-fiction.

It is relevant to add that during this time I came across two separate people, both males, whose general behaviour struck me at the time as a little unusual. In retrospect, some thirty years later, I can now see that they had some of the same awkward traits as I have always had. One was a college student from the group with special needs and learning difficulties, who was always very pleasant to us, but showed a degree of obsessive behaviour. On one occasion he came into the library to fetch a bag of personal possessions which he had left behind, found it was gone, and was about to throw an almighty wobbly. Two or three other members of staff were on hand to help and try to persuade him that we would do our best to help him find it, when just in the nick of time another person returned with it, having taken it away thinking it was his. Both students were very apologetic to each other and to us, and a near-mini-crisis was averted. The other was the husband of a colleague at work whom I met several times, who was my age, and became a good friend. However, the odd veiled comment his wife made to me when he was not around, plus comments by other work colleagues who knew him, and one or two slightly interesting things he did at home which I saw with my own eyes all confirmed my impressions that there was something a little out of the ordinary about him. Like me, he had problems with small talk and the tendency to make rather strange remarks, which I suspect was a result of general unease and the same problems I always had.

That is one reason that I tend to keep quite in conversation, rather than risk making ill-considered remarks off the top of my head which run the risk of making me look or sound foolish. As they say, when in doubt – say nothing. Perhaps it was not always the best strategy. When I was in my teens, my parents – particularly my father – sometimes pulled me up for being taciturn and not getting engaged in conversation with relations who came to stay, giving the briefest of answers to questions which were obviously designed to strike up a conversation. When I was in my late twenties, my niece told me that my aunt had recently remarked somewhat acidly to her that I 'used to write a very good letter, but otherwise I didn't have much to say for myself'. With all due respect, when this aunt was around and in full flow, the rest of the family – not least my father – had little to say for themselves. They had little chance to get a word in edgeways.

Looking back on my earlier life, and knowing what I now do about autism, I can see several of the characteristics that applied to me. From an early age, I tended to take everything and everyone very literally. When my parents used to tell their friends, 'I'll give you a ring,' for years I wondered about this apparent regular exchange of jewellery. Another relevant example was at a school assembly when I was about nine at which the headmaster addressed us, then saw me looking rather puzzled. Looking at me and calling me by name, he asked me directly, 'Has the penny dropped yet?' Having never heard of the phrase, I looked around my feet for this mysterious small coin, while wondering what on earth he was talking about but not having the nerve to ask in front of everyone else. On the other hand, I always understood that 'putting the kettle on' did not mean wearing it as a piece of clothing.

Reverting to schooldays, at the same time I was reasonably good academically at certain subjects, coming top of the form in subjects like English, History and French, and for a while the headmaster nicknamed me 'professor'. When it came to Mathematics and Sciences, I was hopeless. At the time I was quite proud of it and took it as a compliment. Many years later, having read about Hans Asperger's use of the word, I found this rather ironic.

During or very soon after my schooldays I went on a few holidays abroad with my parents, about four times to France and on a couple of occasions to Holland. The former was mainly at my father's suggestion, as he always adored everything French, and latter were largely my choice, as had I persuaded them how lovely it would be to see art galleries in Amsterdam and The Hague. I enjoyed myself, but all the time I was away part of me was longing to be back home. A few years later, I decided that I probably did not want to go abroad again ever, despite the attractions of interesting things to see.

Even then I think I was feeling more comfortable, less insecure, if I stuck to tried and trusted regular routines and familiar places. I passed my driving test at eighteen, but would never take the wheel for long distances on my own (say, anything over fifty miles or so) without somebody to share the duties and navigate me when it was my turn. Stepping forward a little, once I was married, my wife tried to get me to learn to use and love the satnav, with a limited degree of success. Even so it took me a while to feel really comfortable with it, and even then only with places which I knew already to a certain extent. This was more than could be said for taking unfamiliar routes where I would get really stressed out at the likelihood of taking a wrong turning and getting in absolute knots trying to find the correct road again. Whenever I needed to go to London, two hundred miles plus, it would be train or coach every time without a second thought.

It was a failing, a phobia perhaps, which has become more pronounced with age. Another one is an inbuilt resistance to or difficulty to cope with change. However, I am probably not the only computer user who was seized with a feeling of dread ever time Microsoft Word underwent a major makeover or update, and I was confronted with the task of having to relearn where all the regular on-screen functions and drop-down menus were.

I never had a pronounced fear of crowded places. Walking along a busy pavement in Oxford Street on my own never held any fears of me.

With my love of live music, going to gigs, whether part of a crowd or on my own if it was a band I particularly wanted to see, was no problem. On the other hand, for many years I felt very self-conscious about walking into a pub without company.

Another of my traits, certainly since I was an adult, was an aversion to bright lights. Sometimes when I am at home and somebody insists on switching every single light on in the kitchen or living room, I have to put my hand above my eyes as a kind of shield, or leave the room – or just insist on turning a few off and braving the protests of people who do not understand my aversion.

Yet another has been a constant inability to think quickly. I am one of those people who can very rarely answer back, especially if somebody says something wounding or cutting in deadly earnest. It always takes me at least two or three minutes to come back with a suitably assertive reply, by which time of course the moment has long passed. I can at least pride myself on being able to pen a deadly letter or type out a blistering e-mail – but a swift verbal retort would often be so much better. Moreover, at odd times throughout my life someone has asked me a perfectly ordinary question, and I find myself going completely mute, unable to answer for some reason which I can never fathom out. They have generally repeated the question, perhaps thinking I did not hear them the first time round, which has given me a breathing space to say something. It is a minor but perhaps significant characteristic.

Perhaps most important of all was the relationship factor, or rather the lack of relationships. I did sometimes wonder in an undefinable way whether there was something inside me that made me ill-fitted to form one, either long-term or short-term, as there were a couple of brief ones along the way. Most of the time I preferred the company of my cat or cats, and can never remember a time when we did not have at least one in the family. Animals, writes Tony Attwood, practising clinical psychologist and author of several titles on ASD and AS, provide you with unconditional acceptance. The dog is always delighted to see you, the horse seems to understand you and wants to be your companion, while the cat jumps on your lap, and purrs in your company. He suggests that cats are really autistic dogs, so there may be a natural affinity between cats and people with autism and Asperger syndrome.[12]

I had a male cousin, five years younger than me, with whom I have always got on well although we live a considerable distance apart and, not being particularly keen on travel, have only met each other a few times during our lives. He had never married nor had a relationship, or certainly none that the rest of us ever knew about. All the family were convinced that we would be lifelong bachelors. In fact, after my father died, my octogenarian mother had an annexe built on to her house so that I could move in there with one of my sisters and her husband (who lived in the adjoining property next door to us at the time the arrangement was made), living in the house as one happy family together. It only really dawned on me, some time afterwards, that this had been planned as I was probably deemed incapable of looking after myself after she had gone. However, nobody actually spelt it out in so many words.

Let me say that if this had materialised, it would not have been a happy family – but fortunately it was never really put to the test. For when I was in my mid-forties, soon after the start of the new millennium and literally a few weeks after building work on the annexe began, I found love - on the internet. It was not a dating site, but a 'write reviews and get paid per view' affair which had built up a fairly strong online community among its members.

The internet – and again the suggestion emanates from Tony Attwood – has become the modern equivalent of the dance hall in terms of opportunities for young people to meet (and dare I add, even middle-aged). For those with Asperger syndrome it has the advantage in that he or she 'has a greater eloquence in disclosing and expressing thoughts and feelings through typing rather than face-to-face conversation'.[12] In a social context the person is expected to be able to listen to and process the other person's speech, almost always against the distraction of a background of chattering from others (when they can be heard against the music), to reply immediately, and at the same time analyse non-verbal cues like gestures, facial expression and tone of voice. When corresponding on a computer on a one-to-one basis, the person can concentrate on social exchanges without being overwhelmed by the plethora of additional sensory experiences and social signals. I for one can readily identify with that. Much as I revelled in the environment of the regular college discos while a student in London in the 1970s, competing for a space on the dance floor while the DJ served up a healthy high-volume diet of Rolling Stones, Sweet and the like, in retrospect it was not perhaps an ideal setting for serious conversation with the opposite sex.

Of course, a caveat needs to be added in that someone with Asperger syndrome can easily be vulnerable to and being taken advantage of online by false friends. I can vouch for the fact that very positive, lasting relationships can start merely by two like-minded souls living some distance apart, stumbling across each other in cyberspace, discovering a shared interest and watching things gain momentum before they realise it. On the other hand, we are sadly familiar with horror stories where someone strikes up a conversation on Facebook or similar with somebody who appears perfectly pleasant and ordinary online and later turns out to be the very opposite of what they originally seemed, sometimes with grim consequences.

My story was happily very different. My wife-to-be began exchanging opinions and past histories of a sort on the community forum and then by e-mail over the space of several months. Some months later we arranged to meet in person, both with an additional family member in the background. As she later said online, she needed to be sure I was not a mad axeman in sheep's clothing or anything of the kind. To paraphrase a sentence from the last chapter of *Jane Eyre*, 'Reader, I married her', just over a year later. One of my sisters and her husband then announced, with not very good grace, that they were moving to the other end of Europe.

A few months into our engagement, my future wife started to think I was slightly eccentric. Initially she ascribed this to my having lived at home well into middle age with my mother and not having had more than temporary girlfriends in the past. Mercifully, as my previous paragraph will testify, it was not enough to give her serious second thoughts. However, from her point of view the eccentricities gradually became a little more pronounced. At one stage, she wondered aloud whether I might be in the early stages of Alzheimer's. Early fifties is an unusually young age to be displaying any symptoms of dementia, but is not unknown, as the sad experience of the close relation of a family friend proved. My wife and I both had close experience of dementia, in that we each had a parent whose last years had been severely blighted by the condition and who had spent their last few months in care homes as a result.

Maybe it is down to a selective memory, but I have difficulty in remembering them, apart from one which she used to remind me about on a regular basis. For a short time she kept fish in a tank at the end of a kitchen. One day she asked me to put a cup of fresh water in it. I would love to be able to remember the occasion, but she insists that I took her literally and put the whole cup, not just the water inside, in the tank. It may have been my idea of a joke, of course. I will never forget, when I was much younger, my exasperated father writing on the lavatory wall, 'If you use the last sheet – GET ANOTHER ROLL!' - and my brother-in-law helpfully attaching a small bread roll to the holder. I was possibly thinking of that at the time.

Jolly japes apart, serious traits became evident. For example, I did most of the driving during our honeymoon, and on one occasion she told me to 'follow that car over there' in order to get into the correct lane. I followed it a little further than she meant to - no, not as far as the next county boundary, but enough to take us somewhat out of our way. I had no problem with muted indoor lighting, but as already referred to could not manage with what I considered bright lights which everybody else in the family considered normal, and still cannot. Having married into a large family comprising people of all ages from a few months to their seventies, I found it stressful adjusting to a major influx during holiday times. The first time I was sent to go from the kitchen to the adjoining and very crowded living room to ask if anybody would like tea or coffee, perhaps not surprisingly my request went unheard. The second time – well, there was not a second time. I told my wife there was no point in asking, and made it clear why. The only way I could and can still manage with such occasions was - and still is - to remove myself at regular intervals to my study for a little peace and quiet, or go out for a walk, sometimes but not always to the pub, sometimes but not always accompanied by one or two others.

The solitary child who was happy to escape from his own birthday party had become older but to some extent remained the same person inside. I was ill at ease with small children, unless they were unusually quiet and well-behaved. A lot of children, of course, are not – and I did not deal with what any parent will call 'normal' children. My strategy was fight or flight, flight being of course the better option. Being quiet and not talkative by nature, I have often felt uncomfortable in the presence of people who love talking, unless we have common interests. Put me in a group of, say, four adults or more, in which two of them monopolise the conversation. I invariably find it difficult to get a word in edgeways, do not even try to bother to compete, and end up drifting away into my own quiet little world, maybe even nodding off if it is at the end of a long day. That was something I got that from my father.

Talking of whom, I suspect that if anybody had made the suggestion to him that his son had some kind of undefined imprecise mental health issues, he would have dismissed it as nonsense. My mother, whose father had been a GP and who had perhaps considered following in his footsteps if given the opportunity, might have begged to differ. My wife's theory is that, having been broken-hearted after produced one son who died so young, was in perpetual self-denial that she might have given birth to a second who was not quite right. As a result, she thereafter devoted more of her life than she should in covering up for me one way or another. Having an over-protective parent could be very frustrating, to put it mildly.

There were other problems I remember from our first few months of marriage. One was a matter of various hygiene issues that had not mattered much to me, or most of our family, but did to my wife and hers. Another was that she would sometimes ask me to make phone calls on her behalf of a business nature. One that sticks in my mind was some particularly convoluted insurance claim. It was one of several where I had little comprehension of what she was talking about, yet despite her frequently telling me that 'you're no good on the phone', something to which I readily confess, she still asked me to do the work. The only way I could see myself coping with all this information overload was by writing down everything she wanted me to say, so no matter how stressed I would get if stepping outside my comfort zone, I would not forget any important detail. Naturally, I came unstuck if the person on the other end of the line started asking questions. 'Excuse me – can I check …' More often than not, once I had started speaking – or reading out the hastily scribbled script – she would roll her eyes at my having got something wrong (or else left something out as she had forgotten to tell me), before grabbing the handset with an impatient 'Oh, let me do it!' – which would have saved her time in the first place.

Ask me to ring somebody when I know exactly what I am dealing with, I would say. If not, then please make sure I have specific instructions. Otherwise a very stressed (and possibly stuttering), inarticulate caller heading for a verbal train crash on the (telephone) line will be the result. And as for learning to master the basic functions of a mobile phone – let me say that it took some doing. While on an associated subject, later I took a short course in Excel for an ICT (Information Computer Technology) Skills examination. Despite the best efforts of my teacher, I soon feared that I was out of my depth when I failed dismally to grasp a number of the essentials of which I had had almost zero previous experience – and the less said about the exam at the end of it the better.

Was there an element of amnesia in this, I wonder. Having an excellent long-term memory but finding it difficult to recall things which happened only recently is by no means uncommon, particularly in the middle-aged and elderly. There is a widely-held theory that this kind of memory loss, if pronounced and not linked to dementia, can be a symptom of depression. There were times when I became stressed, found it difficult to concentrate, and forgetful to a degree which I found alarming. I would insist on writing things down, partly as I had always found this useful as a safeguard against forgetting them, something which did not always go down well with my wife - whose own short-term memory, by her own admission, was not always perfect.

I would also find myself going into major panic mode on occasion. The worst was one morning when I came to work on the bus and inadvertently left a bag behind containing a large amount of material on a book I was writing. Although I had much of my work in progress backed up on the computer at home, there were also some well-nigh irreplaceable notes which if lost would have caused a major problem. Thankfully – and with the aid of a supportive colleague – once I had realised I was able to phone the bus company who had found everything, enabling me to be reunited with it all a few hours later, but I was thoroughly on edge when I first realised.

I have never been the most practical of people around the house. Fitting a three-pin plug on to an electrical device, changing a light bulb, framing a picture and hanging it on the wall, even painting the wall, are all things I can manage. Changing tap washers, fitting blinds over a window or assembling flat-pack furniture from IKEA are a different matter. I will willingly admit to being quite out of my depth on the first two, though with a little assistance I can sometimes do the latter, after a fashion. Ask me to write a book of up to 90,000 words on something in which I am passionately interested, write a song, words and music, or paint a landscape. Then try and stop me ...

Another stumbling block was my position vis-à-vis small children, in particular an ever-growing brood of step-grandchildren. When I became an uncle at the tender age of eleven, I enjoyed the novelty of sharing the company of my little niece. Further nephews and nieces followed, but as I reached adulthood I somehow lost my way. By the time I reached middle age, I found that any empathy I might have had with a child's mind had gone. This was another characteristic I think I inherited from my father, who told me he was on the whole ill at ease with youngsters, despite having had four himself, and was not ashamed to admit that he was never a hands-on parent who did not have the least desire to hold and cuddle any of us when we were small, although once we got beyond the baby stage and were old enough to take an interest in practical things, that made a difference for the better. I think I also shared his views about strictness and discipline – my wife always said that she thought both my parents were very Victorian in their attitudes – and I admit to having views about upbringing which many people might find out of time in the liberal twenty-first century.

Did my parents tick any of the autism spectrum disorders themselves? Apart from my father's visible withdrawal from us as small babies, and his love of routine – understandable in someone who came from a military family, and whose happiest days were spent as an officer and a pilot in the Royal Air Force during the Second World War – he was probably exempt. My mother's social skills were not of the best, unless they shared her all-consuming interest in all things connected with Dartmoor, and people who did not know her very well sometimes found her quite rude. In her last years, with increasing deafness and general frailty, she became increasingly that way. We had seen it in my father, but in his case the main reason was dementia, something my mother was fortunate not to experience.

Prior to becoming engaged and married, I had been subject to a few bouts of reactive depression, all of which I could put down to as having been triggered by something – normally associated with relationships – which I found very hard to deal with properly. Having always been rather cynical about prescription drugs for such things, I didn't go down that path – I don't think alcohol counts as a prescription drug – and I worked out for myself that dealing with the issues that caused it and moving on were the best cure. Only once did it become bad enough to warrant taking a few days off work, my reason being a heavy cold. It was only about three days or so, and did not extend long enough to warrant a sick note from the doctor.

Fast forward again, about seven years after getting married. My mother had died, which was the cue for some particularly unpleasant legal business involving a close member of the family over which I will hastily draw a veil. All that needs to be said for the purpose of this book was that involved several weeks of trying to obtain the services of a solicitor, much correspondence and a number of meetings with him once we had found the right one, two court appearances, an expensive resolution, much time off work and a very stressful few months which almost certainly contributed to a rather debilitating virus infection. It was perhaps coincidence that this happened in 2008/9, the year the western world caught a rather severe economic cold.

Two years after that, it was crunch time. A period of severe budgeting and financial retrenchment, during which I was almost afraid to look at my bank statements, on paper or online, on a regular basis to see how badly I was overdrawn after the last direct debit, was followed by regime change at my place of work. A new head of service in the department where I worked had recently been appointed, and it soon became apparent that he and one, perhaps two, of the senior supervisory staff were constantly finding fault with my work and attempting to place me on a disciplinary or capability hearing which could result in dismissal. There followed a few increasingly stressful weeks during which I referred myself to the occupational health officer, who was extremely helpful, submitted an official report on the matter, and insisted that I consult my general practitioner at home if matters did not improve. In fact they went from bad to worse.

Over the previous year or two my wife had become increasingly convinced that I was on the autistic spectrum. In a way I owed said staff a vote of thanks, for this became the catalyst for an official referral. As my situation at work became increasingly untenable, I was told to go and see the GP about my constantly falling asleep at work, largely a result of sleeping badly at nights and increasingly exhausted when I turned up next morning. While I did, I spoke to him about the increasing stress and depression issues, and the fact that my wife was convinced I was on the autistic spectrum. At this time I had the feeling that to some extent there was a distinct correlation between the two, and that part of me was not far from meltdown. I had been increasingly in despair about going to work, dreading what unpleasant if not threatening messages would be lurking in my work e-mail box when I logged on to my computer in the office, and even finding it took a great effort to walk in through the front door on arrival each morning. At the same time, I was finding it impossible to look a couple of staff members with whom I was increasingly uncomfortable in the eye – but not the others whom I found unfailingly supportive and helpful, and who recognised in varying degrees something of what was going on.

It was not the first time I had eye contact issues. It was a recurring difficulty while I was growing up, and as a young adult, until I learned the importance of looking somebody in the eye; it did not come naturally to me. Later I realised that, in my mid-forties, I had experienced the same difficulty with a couple of close relatives whom I was finding very hostile. As I was on a forty weeks per year contract, the summer break was looming up, so it took just one week of sick leave to give me seven weeks away from what had suddenly become quite a toxic, increasingly stressful environment.

That same week, my wife completed the report she had been planning for some time to send the GP, a few hundred words in length, mentioning the symptoms and issues which had been giving her concern over the previous few years. In general, she had noticed that it was difficult for me to take on board simple verbal instructions which caused problems with practical tasks at home, that I was prone to paranoia, misreading social situations, and experiencing family difficulties within the family setting, such as not being good with lively step-grandchildren whom I could not (or was not allowed to try and) control, and that friends had noticed this. I completed an online screening questionnaire for autism on which I scored quite highly.

So after an interval of almost two months I returned to work, determined to make a fresh start, and confront the demons head-on. The staff were fully concerned and very understanding. In fairness, I had only had an issue with three of them, one of whom had mercifully left. The two remaining whom I had found it almost impossible to look in the eye when speaking to them a few weeks before were now far more pleasant, now that we had a greater mutual understanding of the underlying situation. As for the others, I had spoken in confidence to two of them. One of them told me that she was very glad I had taken this step as they had been quite concerned, and I think they were relieved to see me back looking more confident and less haunted than before the break.

Just a couple of days earlier I had spoken on the telephone to my previous boss who had retired the year before. We had worked together for over thirty years, and though we had sometimes crossed swords, that was all ancient history by then. During her final few years of working with me she had become increasingly understanding, and on her farewell day we had had a hug and parted as good friends. When I talked to her and apprised her of the situation, she was astonished. She then went on to say that she admitted to knowing very little about ASD, but one thing she knew for certain was that people thus affected always functioned best when they were given very strict instructions for specific tasks with little or no margin for error, and she had rapidly found that she always got the best results from me that way. Armed with this knowledge, which was something I had discovered for myself – if only as confirmation of what I already more or less knew from experience – I told the staff that cheat sheets and the like were the way forward. They were happy to oblige, and the procedure worked well for me.

Another colleague whom I spoke to later, shortly after she had left and started her own business, told me that she could remember I had my own way of doing certain things at work – which was not necessarily the same as everyone else's – and I always did them that way. Looking back on it, I think that even at school and in my earlier years at work, I had a habit of approaching certain tasks my own way. Only at length did I realise that other people's methods were the tried and tested ones which worked far better than my stubbornly independent ones.

By this time I had been referred for an initial assessment with a Locum Consultant Psychiatrist and her assistant. After an interview-cum-consultation with them about two weeks after my return to work (I remember the date distinctly as it was my birthday), they produced a two-page letter to my doctor in which they concluded that there was sufficient evidence to suggest that my longstanding difficulties would justify a more detailed assessment as to whether I had a diagnosis of Asperger's, and they made a referral for me to be seen by the county ADHD/Autism Assessment Service.

About two weeks later, I had a letter from the local NHS Community Mental Health Team, advising me that the Autistic Spectrum Conditions Diagnostic Assessment Service at county level was a new service and that they were still in the process of accepting new referrals, who they would be assessing in due course. As they had just moved into new offices and were having telephones installed, nothing was evidently going to happen in a hurry. Ten months later came another communication to tell me I was at the top of the waiting list and was due to be seen by someone shortly. It was rather frustrating, but there was clearly no quick fix.

About three months after that, the process finally began. I was invited for an initial assessment including an interview and questionnaires to determine whether the difficulties I was experiencing appeared to be consistent with an Autism Spectrum condition, or whether another service would be more appropriate. Over the next couple of months it was followed by two similar meetings, each lasting almost two hours. These sessions included clinical interviews with a Clinical Psychologist and her assistant, attended by myself with my wife present part of the time to add her comments and recollections, as well as psychometric tests designed to detect specific personality traits, and observational assessment to examine my social interaction, social communication and patterns of behaviour, interests and activities. A full developmental history was not feasible as my parents had long since passed away, and my closest remaining relatives with whom I was still in contact were unable to provide anything.

One of my sisters was astonished to hear about the impending diagnosis, as she did not think it at all possible, although her younger son was clearly autistic. She did however tell us after my diagnosis that during childhood she, my other sister and I were once discussing what we wanted to be or do when we grew up. I was aged about five at the time, and I apparently said I was going to work in a library - and I insisted that everyone there was going to be VERY quiet. (My wife thought this was significant, and wished we had known about this earlier). My eldest sister's elder son, who had hinted in the vaguest way possible to my wife when we were engaged that there might be a problem with me, proceeded to tell us very briefly in a letter that, in view of various things I had done or achieved in the past, there was no possibility of my being on the spectrum at all. I remember thinking at the time after I saw what he had written that it was rather inconsistent of him, to say the least.

During these three sessions, my wife and I reported and discussed at some length various problems I had experienced with communication and social interaction, plus restricted interests and behaviour which had been ongoing since childhood. We both brought up examples of incidents I remembered over the years, things my wife had seen which she found unsettling, and also anecdotes which my mother had passed on about me, told with what I assumed were varying degrees of amusement and concern.

Shortly after the third such meeting, the psychologist and her assistant produced a full report about eighteen pages in length, and a brief summary. Their evidence from the assessment, they concluded, indicated 'symptoms which are consistent with a diagnosis of an Autism Spectrum Disorder and meet criteria for a DSM IV diagnosis of Autism.' According to the *Diagnostic and Statistical Manual of Mental Disorders*, this indicated six or more items from the following three criteria:

- Qualitative impairment in social interaction, including marked impairments in the use of multiple nonverbal behaviours such as eye-to-eye gaze, facial expression, body posture, and gestures to regulate social interaction; failure to develop peer relationships appropriate to developmental level; lack of spontaneous seeking to share enjoyment, interests, or achievements with other people, such as by a lack of showing, bringing, or pointing out objects of interest to other people; a dislike of even fear of crowded places

- Qualitative impairments in communication as manifested by at least one of the following: delay in, or total lack of, the development of spoken language (not accompanied by an attempt to compensate through alternative modes of communication such as gesture or mime); in individuals with adequate speech, marked impairment in the ability to make small talk with ease, initiate or sustain a conversation with others; stereotyped and repetitive use of language or idiosyncratic language; lack of varied, spontaneous make-believe play or social imitative play appropriate to developmental level
- Restricted repetitive and stereotyped patterns of behaviour, interests and activities, as manifested by at least two of the following: encompassing preoccupation with one or more stereotyped and restricted patterns of interest that is abnormal either in intensity or focus; apparently inflexible adherence to specific, non-functional routines or rituals; stereotyped and repetitive motor mannerisms (such as hand or finger flapping or twisting, or complex whole-body movements);

persistent preoccupation with parts of objects

The report was accompanied by a post-diagnostic pack including information about help, support, and relevant websites. It concluded with some recommendations, such as an invitation to a group workshop, which would be an opportunity to learn more about the autism spectrum, the challenges people may face and some strategies that may help, as well as an opportunity to meet and share experiences with others who had recently been diagnosed. I was also offered the chance to attend a monthly client network meeting, which would include having a social care assessment within the service to identify any social care needs I might have, and a referral to the Depression and Anxiety Service in order to assist with 'the fairly high levels of anxiety' I appeared to experience. The matter of our concern about my driving (which I shared) was referred to with the recommendation that I discuss it with my GP who could make a referral for a driving assessment if necessary. Perhaps most importantly of all, it was noted that we had learnt that in order to minimise my stress levels it was vital that I was able to leave situations when I needed to, as 'an important and successful strategy for many people on the autism spectrum' which should continue to be encouraged.

So at the age of fifty-eight, my diagnosis was completed.

What were the results? What did I achieve, and what were my feelings? At the risk of sounding either clichéd or idealistic, I think that being armed with the knowledge that I am recognised as being on the autism spectrum has helped me understand and know who, or what, I am. (At this point, cue 'I Am What I Am', from the Broadway musical *La Cage Aux Folles*, as written by Jerry Herman and made famous by Gloria Gaynor; the lyrics are just as appropriate as the title might suggest). For years I lived with a vague sense of feeling that something was not quite right. Once the specialists handed me the diagnosis and a copy of their complete report, in a way it was a kind of relief. My wife and I finally knew what we had long suspected. For the next day or two, both at home and at work, telling management at work (my line manager and the staff at the Human Resources department, both of whom I supplied with a copy of the two-page summary) and my closest friends among my colleagues, I felt that a bit of a burden had been lifted as I now *knew*. I felt less self-conscious, even less guilty, about the various obsessions, aware that I did not have to beat myself up over anything slightly out of the ordinary. Maybe people knew that there was some genuine reason for my preoccupation with quirky trivia, be it vast amounts of not awfully useful knowledge about seventies rock music or, as it would have been at school many years ago, that weird subconscious memorisation of everybody's date of birth.

Did I resent the whole issue not having been nailed, or at least considered, some time before? In a way, I think I did. It might have saved me some years of uncertainty, even spells of depression, had we known earlier. My wife told told me shortly after the diagnosis that she would find it difficult to forgive my late mother for covering up for me for so long and not doing anything about it, when it seemed that she knew - and it would have been in her power to do something towards a referral, a burden which she (my wife) had to shoulder instead. My mother did tell me with a smile shortly after I was engaged that she thought I had not changed in the slightest since I was twenty-one. I thought nothing of it at the time, but later I wondered whether it was a somewhat gilded way of telling me that I had never really grown up, was suffering from arrested development, or something of the kind. However, as I told my wife, it was too late to do anything about it by then.

As for the recommendations in the report, my wife and I realised that my autism was best managed by avoiding stressful situations wherever possible. Being able to remove myself at home from lively family gatherings, including boisterous children - and have the option of not attending them if they took place elsewhere - was vital. The driving was not a problem, as by that time I was usually commuting to and from work by bus. On the rare occasions when my wife and I went to visit family more than, say, two hundred miles away, we kept to an agreement by which I would share the driving on stretches of road with which I was familiar, in order to give her a rest. As much of my activities at home revolved around freelance writing in various non-fiction fields, and as I had spent some time googling a vast amount of information on autism, Asperger syndrome and everything related, I now knew much about the topic and where to look for what I still needed to know. Having been used to spending the odd week or fortnight on my own in the house as an adult some years earlier when my parents were away on holiday, and more recently when my wife was away for a week or so on a family holiday while I was at work, with only a cat or two for company while in the house, I had no genuine need for any support services.

With regard to the offer of follow-up meetings with the psychologist and her assistant, and the opportunity to get together with others at network meetings who had been similarly diagnosed, I turned these down for a couple of reasons. One was because I asked what we would actually do. The verbal answer was 'play games'. I should have asked exactly what games – and I will risk the temptation to make any flippant suggestions – but the idea did not exactly fill me with confidence. In all fairness, I did receive a letter giving me a breakdown of what was involved at a forthcoming meeting. It would be based around 'healthy living', and would include a discussion, followed by 'unstructured time playing games, chatting, etc.' The other was that I did not see any point in going a considerable distance – involving a round trip of around ninety minutes – and trying to fit something into a busy life which could well prove to be valuable time ill-spent. I had the official report, plus several pages of websites to consult for further help and reference, and that was more or less all I needed.

About eighteen months later, I was invited to apply for a personalised alert card (the same size as a banking, debit or credit card) issued by Dimensions for Living, the Devon Foundation for Autism, Asperger syndrome & Related Conditions, marked ATTENTION! POLICE/

EMERGENCY SERVICES: I AM AUTISTIC, to carry around in my wallet with me. It is not a 'get out of jail free', but as the accompanying letter states, to assist me in raising the awareness of my condition that may require 'a different approach' to dealing with me. As of the time of writing, I have not yet needed to show it to anyone, but the feeling of carrying it does provide me with an additional safety net, even if only a small one.

My wife and I have a mutual friend, a musician, about fourteen years younger than me, who is autistic. He has marked communications with speech, and anybody meeting him for the first time will immediately be aware that there is something not quite right, especially if they try to hold a conversation with him. One interesting thing about him, I have observed, is that he has had a tendency to lose things, sometimes in our car or in a bag just outside our gate, sometimes not. As far as we can see, losing anything never seems to make him panic. If I lose something important – which I am glad to say happens rarely – I become really stressed, as if it is almost the end of the world.

I have learned how to live with the conditions, not feel guilty about having them or about not going out of my comfort zone for the sake of it. Trying to contain and live with obsessive quirks, such as subconsciously counting steps on staircases or feverishly check my bag at least once or twice before I go to work in the morning or leave in the afternoon at least twice at intervals, to ensure I have not forgotten or – heaven forbid, lost - anything really vital, is part and parcel of the baggage, something to be accepted. I regularly have mild little flashbacks about things that I did, or that happened to me, in the past and which somehow did not make sense at the time, but which do now. I still get worried about forthcoming events which are liable to be taxing, panic if I cannot remember computer passwords, or find certain important objects – like my keys, which I dropped in the garden one Friday evening and spent a frantic few hours searching for until I saw them about midnight five hours later - and have a tendency to stutter when I get really stressed. I mentioned above that some people on the spectrum are good at keeping calm in a crisis while others around them go into panic mode; sometimes I can, on other occasions I might be the first to go to pieces.

I still have problems with sensory overload, taking in new things like practical instructions on how to use gadgets, and have to write the important things down before I forget what I have been told. On occasion when somebody is explaining something convoluted to me, I have to ask them to go through it again more slowly, not because I have not heard properly or not paying attention (I have heard and listened to them, honestly), but because I realise I am not grasping or understanding what I am being told and my brain needs more time to process it properly. It may not always go down well with the other person – but that can hardly be helped. If I am going anywhere unfamiliar on my own for the first time, whether on foot, by car or by public transport, I need to research it thoroughly, even to the point of printing out a basic plan or road map to take in my pocket and paying a preliminary visit first in good time if I can, largely as a sign of reassurance that 'all will be well'. (As my father used to tell me, 'time spent in reconnaissance is never wasted'.) I am still no good at small talk and feel slightly intimidated by those who can talk effortlessly for England, whether in person or on the phone. My wife now accepts that it is best to let her deal with telephone queries on matters that I do not understand. Above all, I still experience times of 'being in a dark place' – never more so than when I was notified that I was 'at risk' in my job and found myself under some pressure to accept 'voluntary' redundancy. But I think I can take these things in my stride rather more easily than before.

*Kerry, a former line manager at my place of work, kindly contributed the following.*

I was first introduced to Jon by the Library Manager, when starting in my new role in the Library. Unbeknownst to me, the position I had taken involved line management of three members of staff. I had found this out just two hours before this encounter, and I was now meeting one of the people I would have to support for the next couple of years, so I swallowed my anxiety and summoned some confidence.

Jon introduced himself with a smile and shook my hand firmly. We had a brief chat, before I went through to the office to start my training. The first thing that struck me about Jon was how well-spoken he was. His idiolect was formal; almost regal, and stance was marked by his arms folded across his chest.

'I'm surprised Jon shook your hand,' said my line manager, as the door to the office closed. I was perplexed; a handshake is surely the best introduction in a work setting between future colleagues, and he seemed perfectly pleasant, if not a little formal; so, out of curiosity, I pressed her for a reply.

'I'm not breaking any confidences by informing you that Jon has high-functioning Asperger's Syndrome,' she replied. Having worked with several Autistic people in the past, I heaved a sigh of relief. This was more familiar territory than management!

In the first couple of months of my role, I quickly established a rapport with Jon through a mutual love of 70's music and my fascination with his keen abilities as a writer. It took some time to figure out how Jon ticked which we trialled with different tasks, with varying success.

As advised by the Library Manager, I would give Jon instructions, and allow him to write them down step by step. This is where I learned the importance of 'say what you mean', as unless the directions were explicit, Jon would work with what he had on paper, until told otherwise: warts and all.

Eventually, Jon and I had a frank discussion about his workload and something clicked in our working relationship. I realised that Jon was a fantastic worker; in fact, if you ever need your library moved, shelved or otherwise, give him a call; but in trying to capture the details of a task by writing them down, he was missing small details that would occur in practice, but were nonetheless pivotal to an accurate job.

From that point onwards, I changed my approach. If I asked Jon to do something, I would give him some basic instructions, which he could annotate, and we would do a few working examples together, until he had perfected the routine. Jon only needed to be shown once or twice and could complete reams of lists in a short time frame, which was absolutely essential to the running of the library.

Jon was the perfect example of how an individual diagnosed with Asperger's Syndrome is as an asset in the workplace. He contributed to staff meetings in a way that other members of staff could not, which I believe came from his preference for structure and routine, resulting in several improvements to Library operations. He would keep meticulous records which could always be traced back, and despite his own feelings on counter service, he had an excellent customer service manner.

Of course, there were obstacles to overcome, but no more than with other members of staff. I greatly valued Jon as a member of the team, and always saw his contributions as positive. I feel that we achieved a good working relationship over the years we worked together, which we shaped together, into a mutual respect and understanding of one another. Although Jon and I no longer work together, we keep in touch, and I believe that part of the reason that this friendship has continued, is due to the efforts we

made whilst working together, and for all the
things I learned about the condition along the
way.

# ... and yours?

Health professionals, whether general practitioners or psychologists, will contend that probably everybody shares at least one personal characteristic with people on the spectrum. They also strongly advise against self-diagnosis. Anybody can read a book, an article, or even find a quiz or list online which apparently does the job for them. A recent school of thought suggests that Asperger's has become 'a trendy disease' to assume people have in order to explain social disaffection or act as an alibi for eccentricity. People who are genuinely struggling with the suspicion that they are affected, or whose partners or families seriously believe they are, are advised to consult their doctor.

At this stage, I can do no better than to acknowledge and briefly summarise the step-by-step recommendations of the National Autistic Society.

If you think you or a close family member might be autistic, you (or he/she) can always take one of the online tests available, but these do not guarantee accuracy, and any intelligent person can generally answer the questions in such a way as to give the answer they would like it to provide. I am one of many people who went through much of my life on the spectrum without knowing it, only aware that somehow I did not 'fit in'. Some people find it increasingly hard to cope and need to be sure for their own peace of mind (in which case a self-diagnosis might or might not be sufficient), while others such as myself may suddenly find themselves up against a potential crisis on the horizon that makes action imperative. It is only right to add at this point that autism and Asperger syndrome vary widely from person to person, so a genuine formal diagnosis provided by a multi-disciplinary diagnostic team, a psychiatrist or a clinical psychologist with experience in diagnosing autism, is advisable.

The first step is to make an appointment with your GP, ensuring that this is the only issue about which you are seeing him or her. If you bring the subject up in the course of consultation about another health issue ('oh, and before I forget to mention it, doctor, I think I might be autistic ...'), it will probably not be given due attention or treated with the priority it deserves. Although it is not essential, should your parents have passed away, if you have official support in the form of a short written report from your partner or another family member explaining the reasons why they or you think you are on the spectrum, or if they can accompany you to explain why, this will be helpful to everybody concerned. It goes without saying that you will probably have difficulty in talking in measured terms about your symptoms, and at the very least it would make it easier to have somebody to back you up and reinforce the case. Sometimes, a person close to you can – and often does – perceive and explain the problems better, in clearer detail and with arguably more confidence than you can yourself. Such a person can provide more accurate validated evidence.

An example has been given by Tony Attwood, citing the case of an adult referred for assessment who was asked about his friends when he was a child and whether other children would visit him at home. He said that they did, implying a degree of popularity and friendship. His mother confirmed that children did indeed visit, but not to play with her son, rather to play with his toys while he shunned their company, amusing himself on his own with a Lego set in the bedroom.[12] Once you have been referred, there will be no further active involvement from your GP, although he or she will doubtless receive a copy of any subsequent report as a matter of courtesy and interest, as mine did.

The Society recommends that it may be helpful to take along a copy of their guidance for GPs, and tell him or her about the relevant guidelines on autism recognition and referral that should guide their decision. Personally I would have thought this might have verged on the insulting. Would you hand the barman at your local a sheet of printed instructions on how to pour your pint of beer or glass of wine? However, the official view is that not all GPs will have an in-depth knowledge of autism, and if this is the case with yours, the guidelines will help. At the least, they need to be aware of NICE (National Institute for Health and Care Excellence) Guideline 142, which covers diagnosing and managing suspected or confirmed autism spectrum disorder (autism, Asperger syndrome and atypical autism), in people aged eighteen and over, aims to improve access and engagement with interventions and services, and the experience of care, for people with autism, and be aware of the statutory guidance published to ensure the implementation of the adult autism strategy and telling local authorities, NHS bodies and NHS Foundation Trusts what actions should be taken to meet the needs of people with autism living in their area, requiring a clear diagnosis pathway for adults. In my case, though, my GP was well aware of what to do next, having been made aware beforehand through my wife's written report, and knew the steps to take with regard to referral as well as the details of diagnostic services in our local area.

You will probably be referred to a diagnostic service, such as a clinic or assessment centre, in your local Clinical Commissioning Group area (in England), your Health Board area (in Scotland), your Local Health Board area (in Wales), or your Health and Social Care Trust area (in Northern Ireland). You can be referred to a service outside your area, but as this will cost more, your local NHS commissioning body might question why you need to go there, or whether you really need a diagnosis. Private diagnosis is always possible if you can pay for one, but you may find that local service providers such as social services will not accept these and insist that the job is done by the NHS diagnosis.

In the unlikely event that your GP decides not to refer you for a diagnosis, you have every right to ask why. Should you feel uncomfortable discussing their decision then and there, you can request a second appointment to discuss the matter, or even ask if you can see another GP at the surgery. As a last resort, if you want to complain about the referral or the diagnostic service you received, you can make an official complaint in writing to the local authority.

For the diagnostic assessment, you will probably be given an appointment with a psychiatrist, clinical psychologist or multi-disciplinary team. There is no standard waiting time, as it depends largely on the availability of qualified personnel available to see you. As mentioned above, for my initial referral I had a six-week interval, and received the report about a month later advising that I would be seen by the Diagnostic Assessment Service at county headquarters. This was still in the process of being set up at the time and I was just one name on a list, hence a slightly unsettling wait of about sixteen months after that. None of the diagnoses are medical examinations, as there is no need or requirement for a physical examination or any samples, such as blood.

For the purposes of the diagnosis, a person will usually be assessed as having had persistent difficulties with social communication and social interaction and restricted and repetitive patterns of behaviours, activities or interests, including sensory behaviour, or difficulty processing everyday information, since early childhood, to the extent that these limit and impair everyday functioning. There will probably be a series of questions about your developmental history from when you were a young child about language, play and cognition, and one of the tests similar to those which can be found online to see how high or low your score is.

Sometimes the diagnosticians will tell you whether or not they think you are autistic on the day of the final assessment consultation, or they may send or bring you the report in person at a later stage. It will probably say that you present a particular autism profile, such as an Asperger syndrome or Pathological Demand Avoidant profile. If the diagnostic report proves difficult to read or understand in places, you are welcome to contact the diagnostician to talk through any parts that you find unclear, but alternatively you may find that looking up anything that requires clarification online is more straightforward and convenient.

Occasionally people go through the process to be told they are not autistic after all. If this happens to you, you may be relieved, or alternatively (and more probably) find you have received a diagnosis you do not agree with. You can seek a second opinion, which either means going back to your GP to explain that you are not satisfied and would like to be referred elsewhere, or pay for a private assessment. (The Society does not give an estimate as to how much this is likely to cost, so draw your own conclusions). If you go for a second assessment, remember that it may reach the same conclusion as your first. Should you be diagnosed as autistic, you may have many questions to ask. You might be wondering how you can find out more about your condition, meet other autistic people, or access services and support. Some people may require post-diagnostic support, while others feel that having the diagnosis is basically enough.

Widely different reactions have been reported to diagnosis. Most suggest that it has been a very positive experience, often one of relief that people on the spectrum know for certain that they have the same problems as many others, that there is a genuine reason why they feel apart from much of the human race, and that it provides an explanation of why they were different to everybody (or nearly everybody) else in some ill-defined way.

On the other hand, there are those who may feel angry at the delay in their being diagnosed late in life. 'The System' has left them unrecognised for so long, and they may experience a sense of frustration, even despair at how their lives might have been easier had the diagnosis been confirmed long before, or for the 'wasted years' during which they felt misunderstood, inadequate, stigmatised or rejected.[12]

Gillan Drew was diagnosed at the age of twenty-eight. His mother watched a programme about a boy with Asperger Syndrome who seemed in every way identical to how he had been in childhood. After doing some research into the subject, she realised that he fulfilled all the diagnostic criteria. The psychiatrists she contacted were reluctant to send him to a specialist as they were adamant he did not have it. When she eventually persuaded them, a specialist told her within minutes that he was definitely on the spectrum. He subsequently wrote of his experiences and of a period of adjustment during which, he says, 'you question everything you thought you knew, which can leave you feeling confused and insecure'.[13] He maintains that it is not uncommon to deny the diagnosis, and leave people who are affected feeling unsure of who they should tell, who to go to for help, and what they might need to deal adequately with the condition.

Some diagnostic teams and professionals will offer you follow-up services after diagnosis, and should be able to answer your questions and point you towards support services if you require them, but not all. Support does not automatically follow diagnosis, and if you are capable of leading a fully independent life, as are many people on the spectrum. But having a formal diagnosis means that you are more likely to be able to access services and claim any benefits to which you may be entitled. Anybody who is caring for an adult is in theory entitled to a carer's assessment, while disability benefit can be paid if you have care needs or mobility differences. The rules and conditions are far from straightforward, and legislation is always subject to change, so it is recommended that you refer to www.autism.org.uk/benefits for the most up to date information. This naturally applies only to those on the spectrum who have difficulty in living independently.

If you do not qualify for benefits, the advantages of an assessment and diagnosis are that at the very least they will help you to understand why you may experience certain difficulties and what you can do about them. Sometimes it may correct a previous misdiagnosis, such as schizophrenia, and thus mean that any mental health issues can be better addressed. On occasion it can be difficult to make a diagnosis of autism where there are severe mental health issues, or where someone is receiving treatment. It is your responsibility to ensure that the appropriate people at your place of work have a printed copy of the diagnosis. They are legally required to make any necessary reasonable adjustments, treat you with understanding and be aware of any allowances which may need to be made for you, and you are entitled to expect these.

I have read of adults who have been diagnosed in their forties and said afterwards that it was not about seeking support, which they discovered was virtually non-existent, but about seeking a better understanding of their own identity. It helped them come to terms with their own limitations and their family to understand the issues better. Some required a formal diagnosis to overcome problems in their marriages, relationships or, as in my case, the workplace.

One in his early forties said that although he had managed to function quite well, with a career and a family, nobody else really knew how much anxiety he was masking as he had previously felt 'a bit like an alien in the world'. Others, particularly those in middle age, may not find it necessary, and can obtain understanding, enabling self-management by reading up on autism and perhaps talking to others. On the other hand, there are cases of those who are diagnosed late in life and have been promised follow-up help or specialist counselling 'at a later stage' as soon as funding became available – and were subsequently kept waiting indefinitely, much to their frustration.

It is by no means unusual for people on the spectrum to have gone through their entire working lives without a diagnosis of autism, yet always feeling that somehow they do not quite fit in, or have been mildly disadvantaged yet without fully understanding the reason why. They have learned to cope with life in their own ways, although not without difficulty. Some of them might be married or living with a partner, and have families or successful careers, while others may be more isolated and find things more of a struggle, or perhaps living with an over-protective elderly parent who has managed to cover up for them – in which case, once that parent dies, they could face severe personal issues once they are on their own. It is up to you whether you decide to seek a diagnosis. Some people are happy to remain self-diagnosed, but as the foregoing demonstrates, there are advantages in an official diagnosis. I speak as one of many for whom it worked well, and looking back on it, am very relieved that I was sent on that journey. (And not just because this book you are reading is one of the results).

Not long ago I read a comment somewhere saying that just because autistic people want a diagnosis does not mean they want special treatment. It means they want to know they are not mad or mentally deficient, and there is a sound reason for why some people are different. All they are asking for is simple acknowledgement and recognition of the fact. For too long they have been regarded at school, at work or anywhere else with a lack of comprehension at best, amusement at worst, been made to feel like outcasts, because they are not the same as everybody else.

# Autism, Asperger syndrome, and employment

Young adults who have not already reached the stage of employment require support of a different kind. As people with Asperger syndrome often have great skills and expertise or specialised knowledge in a particular field or subject area, this can be invaluable in certain lines of business, and more than compensates for what might seem to others a slightly and totally justifiably eccentric personality. Those who are embarking on student life at college or university will need to disclose any diagnosis in order to ensure that appropriate support and guidance will be forthcoming where necessary.

So when it comes to applying for a job, should you be honest about your autism or Asperger syndrome? Yes – and no.

The results of a survey in *Autism Spectrum News* in 2011 revealed that between 15% and 25% of people with Asperger syndrome work full-time. Is there ever a right time for aspiring employees to disclose their diagnosis and increase or ruin their chances of getting the job? It is generally seen as a major impediment in joining the workforce as it affects behaviour in ways that are not often understood by those who are not familiar with it. As those with Asperger tend to take things literally, no matter what the context, it is difficult for them to interpret subtle social cues, such as tone of voice, facial expression, and body language. Appearing to be emotionally flat and expressionless, highly focused on detail and sensitive to noises and interruptions, they have problems in coming across well and failing to shine in job interviews, and risk being seen by members of the interviewing panel as unintentionally unfriendly if not downright rude.

There is no right or wrong answer as to whether applicants should or should not disclose a diagnosis of Asperger's in a job interview. Some people thus affected can make a good impression in a short conversation, albeit with effort, and they may choose not to disclose their diagnosis until and unless it becomes absolutely necessary. Others may be anxious that their flat demeanour and problems with interpreting social signals will make a bad impression and cost them a job for which they are well suited. They may wish to disclose their diagnosis at an early stage so the employer will know not to interpret their manner the wrong way.

As a rule, though, it is considered not advisable to disclose a diagnosis in a covering letter unless it is likely to be perceived as an asset by the employer. People with Asperger's tend to perform well at jobs which requiring close attention to detail and meticulous focus, and some employers might regard a person with Asperger syndrome as just right for such work. When disclosing a diagnosis in an interview, therefore, there are two approaches. One is to give a full, concise disclosure of the diagnosis, its likely effects on performance in the job, and any accommodations the employer could make. The other is to say as little as possible but to cover the main points. If making a full disclosure, it is necessary to be as concise and clear as possible and avoid any unnecessary details. Employers in Britain and America should be conversant with the basic issues, and are legally required to make reasonable accommodations for employees with autism spectrum disorders under employment legislation with regard to disabilities and discrimination.

Reading through online forums produces widely differing views, as ever. Some people suggest that on rare occasions a diagnosis can be an advantage, but on the whole, the ignorance of 'normal people' suggests that disclosure is unwise. It is best not mentioned in a covering letter or resumé. The only time an employer should know about a disability or health problem is if it would prevent an applicant from doing the job fully, and if that is the case, he or she is best advised not to apply for the job in the first place. There is no reason to tell employees about this prior to their offering the job, and even in the position it is best not to disclose a diagnosis unless absolutely necessary in order to avoid discrimination.

While sorting through letters of application and CVs, the first priority of employers is to whittle down the number of interviewees. The ethical implications of not hiring somebody on the spectrum are unlikely to be at the top of their list, unless they take the equal opportunities or positive discrimination ethos really seriously. An employee who is disabled or has a diagnosis of potential mental health issues might be viewed as being more hassle than he or she is worth, and on these grounds would be among the first to be eliminated. Some organisations state clearly on job advertisements that they are 'an equal opportunities employer', but even then it is often deemed as well not to make a disclosure unless absolutely necessary. Diagnoses are sometimes misunderstood, much as everyone would like to think that equal opportunities employers will have due sensitivity towards the issue. A few people go so far as to maintain that all organisations in theory say that they are 'equal opportunities', but in practice not so. Unless a job is specifically looking for people on the spectrum, it is best not to disclose it.

Some people maintain that a disclosure of diagnosis should never be made for any reason unless not to do so would be a direct and immediate lie to a direct question, or unless an applicant really wants to 'weed out bigoted workplaces'. Bringing up specific weaknesses and concerns, such as not being good at small talk or socialising, is a fine art and can perhaps be introduced gently into an interview, should the opportunity arise. But using the a- word is often considered an absolute no-no, except on an application for disability benefits.

Others see it as being useful to mention their diagnosis in the cover letter of each job they apply for, so that employers know why they do not converse well during an interview. They realise that this can discourage people from hiring them, but they think it the only way to be honest and let people know that their below-average conversational skills are no reflection on their ability to do the job.

Although there has been a change in attitudes in recent years for the better, mental health issues are still not always fully understood. If employers think that a diagnosis is likely to affect someone's ability to make a success of the job, they are allowed to – or do subconsciously, anyway - discriminate on the basis of expected job performance but not disabilities. Would-be employees do not want to give them a reason for discrimination, but at the same time they may already be discriminating against them as a result of unsatisfactory demeanour during the interview. 'Putting a label' on their behaviour is one way of getting round that concern. Arguably, bearing in mind that autistic people can improve their verbal and non-verbal demeanour with training, a better solution is for applicants to try and focus on their interviewing skills and practice interviewing.

A recent study points out that part of hiring people involves interviews, which can in itself cause problems if the person is not comfortable around new people and with a mix of social difficulties. But if more workplaces were autism aware, people on the spectrum may be employed as the workplace will know how to deal with having a member of staff who has been diagnosed.[10]

When I was in my early twenties, I applied for a job and felt I interviewed quite well. Although I was not offered it, the same employer had an almost identical vacancy in the same department some ten months later and contacted me to ask whether I would like to be considered for the post. I was accordingly interviewed again, and one of the two people who had been on the panel the first time round was there again. (On the second occasion, I noticed that he did not smile at all, in contrast to the first – and smoked incessantly. Only later did I learn that he was having major personal issues at the time. The other panel member asked nearly all the questions). I felt that the second interview did not go as well as the first, and that I was not at my best. Towards the end, the aforementioned member of the panel said that I had been applying for several jobs, and did I ever wonder why I was being turned down. 'I don't think I come across well at interviews,' I told him. After being sent to wait in the next room for a few minutes. I was called back. He told me that one of the other candidates had been excellent, and by rights they should be offering her the post. I obviously wanted it, and I was absolutely right in admitting that I did not interview well, 'but we've looked beyond that.' This was in 1977, long before the days that autism and 'we are an equal opportunities employer' entered general parlance.

# Does autism run in families?

Research suggests that there may be a hereditary factor, and that it is or might be handed from one generation to the next. Bearing in mind that our willingness as a whole to acknowledge mental health issues is a fairly recent phenomenon, and that the whole issue of autism is likewise still in its infancy, I think we can conclude that the jury is out on this one. I have however read enough to suggest that it seems to run in families. I have a nephew whom I like and respect greatly, and who has Obsessive Compulsive Disorder, and I had an elder brother who died at the age of four before I was born. My mother never talked about him to me, although in her eighties, when I was engaged, she did open up to my wife-to-be about him a little. It was apparent that he had Down's Syndrome, at a time – the 1940s – when such things were not really recognised, that he probably had epilepsy, and that he went deaf and blind during his short life, and that had he been born two or three days later he might have been saved – although whether he would have been cured of his conditions, we cannot say.

Several years before my mother died, my mother was turning out some papers and gave me a handful to put on the bonfire. Among them were some of the last letters from her father-in-law, who died at the age of seventy-two in 1947, several years before I was born. One written a few days before he died, when he plainly knew that his time was almost up, included some pompous remarks about how disappointed he was that his only living grandson, my brother, was 'not going to make the grade'. My mother must have found this incredibly hurtful, so no wonder she wanted me to set light to it.

This grandfather had something of a reputation among the family as a bully. It was occasionally let slip that his first wife, my grandmother, died in her early sixties in a nursing home, with alcoholism being a contributory cause. I remember my father talking to me from time to time about his brothers, he being the youngest of four, and I remember two quite well. The youngest was killed in 1940 during the Second World War. But he almost never spoke to me about his father, and never about his mother. Some years after he died, we discovered that he had had two cousins living not far from us, and we were never aware of their existence until long after they had died. He never mentioned them either. It was as if he had cut himself off from most of his family for some reason.

I am aware that this has gone a little off-topic, and I apologise. It was not meant to turn into a veiled rant against the history of a somewhat dysfunctional family. However, to steer things back to the subject, my wife always suspected, as did I with hindsight, that my mother was desperate not to face up to the possibility that her first son had 'not made the grade' as her father-in-law coldly put it, and that there was

something not quite right about her second son
- me - as well.

Coming back to the subject, experts generally agree that the genes for autism are linked to those that confer a talent for grasping complex systems and concepts, such as computer programs and scientific theories. In recent years it has been noted that mathematicians, engineers and physicists tend to have a relatively high rate of autism among their relatives.

At the same time, as we have become increasingly aware of the condition, and adults are being diagnosed increasingly as a result of their children having just gone through the same process. It happened to Lynne Watkins, who only discovered - or one might say realised - that she was autistic at the age of forty-one after her two small sons were identified as being on the spectrum, and she recognised the same traits in herself. When the younger one was a baby, she was afraid to look him in the eye as his intense gaze unnerved her, made her shudder and feel sick. If she was having a bath, she needed to turn the children's toy ducks around so they were not looking at her. She also felt a similar panic when somebody in sunglasses approached her, as the lenses resembled big staring eyes. These last two symptoms were characteristic of the trouble with eye contact experienced by many.

Her sons were identified as autistic before starting school. When she was initially told by the specialists that they had trouble with eye contact, did not play with other children and 'loved routines', such as looking forward to their regular swimming lessons every week and experiencing a tremendous feeling of shock if they were cancelled, and their anxiety with unfamiliar places, it sounded like perfectly normal behaviour to her.

Only later did it occur to her that she shared some of their linguistic and social difficulties, albeit in milder form, and that the traits pointed out to her by the specialist were things she understood perfectly from her own experience. The boys were both at the low-functioning end of the spectrum. The elder could construct basic sentences and had attended college but had minimal social skills, and lived semi-independently in his mother's home, while they younger had never developed speech or a full understanding of the outside world, would lash out if distressed by a change to his routine or sensory overload, and had been in full-time residential care from the age of eleven. Their mother had Asperger syndrome, loved routines and patterns, hated crowded or unfamiliar places and struggled to make friends. In spite of it she went to college, married (and divorced), raised a family, had an exceptional memory and organisational skills, ran her own craft business, and also wrote a book on autism. In spite of that she admitted to an acute sense of missing out, and longing for the friendship that comes from shared jokes and mutual understanding. She also suffered from what she called 'tunnels of hell'. If a friend dumped her or if she found herself in a stressful situation, 'my mind torturously repeats all the put-downs people have ever said to me. All these hurtful sentences come back and shout incessantly in my brain for 24 hours a day except for a few hours' sleep. The only way I can stop them is to play my iPod at full volume.'

At length she confided in her GP her feeling that she thought she might be autistic. When he asked if she did anything 'odd', she said it was hard to give him an answer that because obviously she did not see herself doing anything unusually. She asked if she could be referred to the consultant psychiatrist who had assessed her sons, and her diagnosis was accordingly confirmed. To her it was more a relief than a shock. She likened it to being on a red road of life and she used to think everyone was on the red road. 'Then gradually I've discovered everyone else is on the blue road. It runs parallel but it's not the same road. Now I know that, it's easier for me. I talk more nowadays and feel more confident.'[2]

Another parent who followed the path of his children was a former teacher aged forty-eight, who was diagnosed in 2013, two years after his ten-year-old son. His eldest daughter, two years older, was diagnosed with a high-functioning form of autism a few months ago. When his wife started reading up on autism and noticed the many personality traits shared by father and son, including a difficulty in reading facial expressions and body language and aversion to loud noises and social situations. She told her husband – and suddenly it all made sense. He realised he had always found it a struggle to understand what other people were talking about, and while happy to sit and listen, small talk made no sense to him. 'It sounds terrible but I feel no emotional connection with other people. Joining conversations and recognising social cues are a nightmare.' His wife has learned to guide her husband and their children through the potential minefields. While admitting that he can bore people endlessly about military history unless she stops him, he recognises that he has come to terms with managing the problem, improving in a social capacity, and has become less withdrawn than he was formerly. One negative side is what he perceives as a lack of support for autistic adults in his local area, near Glasgow.

This is a perception shared by a forty-one-year-old professional photographer, who asked to be assessed after he realised he felt similar disengagement, confusion and anxiety to that of his four-year-old autistic daughter. He was advised by doctors that although he had Asperger syndrome, it was not worth seeking a diagnosis as there was so little help for autistic adults. He disputed the verdict, maintaining that he had a right to be diagnosed, as being the father of a daughter thus affected had 'made me realise who I am.'

Reading through articles in newspapers and magazines, and postings online, makes it clear that these cases are by no means exceptional. As a member of teaching staff at the college where I worked for many years told me when I was initially aware that I might be on the spectrum, 'you are not alone'.

Something must be said about a perceived lack of support. This naturally depends on everybody's situation and needs. If you are diagnosed as autistic, and you have the post-diagnostic report on paper to prove it, you are entitled to whatever assistance you feel you need and want. Even if you are capable of leading a more or less normal life and career with, shall we say, very minor adjustments, you have a right to be recognised as such by family, friends, colleagues and line managers in the workplace. Your family will accept that allowances need to be made, as will senior staff at work as they are required by law. To do otherwise could mean that they are guilty of discriminating against you, and in this day and age it would be an exceptionally hard-hearted boss to treat you unfairly – apart from which, he or she would be breaking the law. There have been cases of people who have had to leave work against their inclinations, receive a diagnosis and later rejoin the workforce.

One man in his late fifties had a son who was diagnosed with Asperger syndrome at the age of six. He recalled that as a child he was odd, found it agony to mix socially, and through his teenage and much of his adult life did his best to avoid it. Eye contact was also a problem. Since the birth of his son, through curiosity, he had tried various DIY autism tests although they always proved negative. He wondered whether his son's condition might be explained in part by the fact that he was an older father, in his forties, when the son was born.

With greater self-awareness of autism in adults, there has inevitably been a negative side. A new school of thought has regrettably materialised in which some people maintain that too many in this day and age are encouraged by the media, and perhaps perceptions of political correctness, to see themselves as victims by our society. To this, the clear answer is that people who think, and then know, they are on the spectrum, do not regard themselves as victims. All they are doing is gaining a greater understanding of themselves, recognising the problem and dealing with it the most satisfactory way possible. One astonishing – not to say unsympathetic - comment that I saw on an online forum asserted that women seemed to revel in 'victim' status nowadays, asking 'why take responsibility for your actions when you can claim that you are disadvantaged?' Thankfully it had provoked a fierce response to the effect that people who have been diagnosed are not seeking sanctuary by making false claims on behalf of themselves but genuinely have a real condition suffered in various degrees by millions. Another remark I have read on similar lines is that diagnoses create their own victims, 'and people can cling to them tenaciously'.

One woman posted on a forum that she was convinced her husband had Asperger syndrome, although not the diagnosis. He lacked empathy, or at least the ability to demonstrate it, and tact, something which on occasion got him into trouble at work as his frustrations led him to say something he would have done better to keep to himself. He had a history of being bullied badly at school, and in adult life he still struggled to form friendships. While suffering from depression, he never hid behind it as an excuse to miss work or fulfil his responsibilities. If he had a formal diagnosis, his wife believed, it would almost certainly help them both to understand him more and learn better how to cope with life. In conclusion she said that it was not used as an excuse or as a reason to be treated as a victim, but merely a way of personal understanding, and allowing others to achieve a better understanding of him and why he sometimes behaved the way he did.

Another view is that while everyone now acknowledges that autism clearly exists, the explosion in diagnosis rates during the last few years might be in part a reflection of how inward-looking we have become as we hide behind our digital devices and retreat into our virtual worlds, and a good excuse for self-centred behaviour. Again, this I find rather contentious, to say the least, and quite probably emanating from someone who is not on the spectrum themselves and does not know anybody who is.

# Autism: the pioneers

**Dr Leo Kanner** (1894-1981), born in Austro-Hungary, was a psychiatrist and physician who practised in Germany before moving to America in 1924. In 1930 he was appointed to develop the first child psychiatry clinic in the United States at Johns Hopkins Hospital, Baltimore, where he became the Chief of Child Psychiatry three years later. He was the first physician in America to be identified as a child psychiatrist. In 1935 his first textbook, *Child Psychiatry*, became the first work in the English language to focus on the psychiatric problems of children.

In 1943 he published a paper, *Autistic Disturbances of Affective Contact*, in which he described the results of a study, carried out over five years, of eleven children who were very intelligent but had largely withdrawn from social interaction by the age of two, showing 'a powerful desire for aloneness' and 'an obsessive insistence on persistent sameness'. The fundamental issue of this disorder, he asserted, was their inability to relate to people and objects in an ordinary way from birth. He also noted that many of them were delayed in their speech, that those who were verbal tended to use speech in peculiar ways, such as regular repetition of phrases, that their behaviour was governed by an anxious and obsessive desire for sameness, and that this resulted in repetitive actions, such as their verbal utterances, and limited spontaneous activity. At the same time many of them had very retentive memories, and found it easy to learn favourite songs or poems, lists of animal and botanical names, and random facts. He named the condition 'early infantile autism', the last word being from 'auto', Greek for 'self'. It was his belief that there was a biological reason for the condition, which appeared very early in life and could therefore not be blamed on outside causes, so they must have been born without social instinct.

**Hans Asperger** (1906-80), an Austrian doctor, was best known for his early studies on mental disorders, especially in children, and as a result of his pioneering work on autism spectrum disorders, Asperger syndrome was named after him. In his own childhood, he had had some of the symptoms that he would later detect in others.

The definition of autistic psychopathy that he published in 1944 was similar to a definition published in 1926 by a Russian neurologist, Grunya Sukhareva. He identified in four boys a pattern of behaviour and abilities including lack of empathy, problems in forming friendships, one-sided conversations, a tendency to become single-minded in what they were doing, and clumsy movements. Because of the detail they would go into while describing their particular interests, he called them 'little professors'. Some of the children he had identified as being autistic were particularly knowledgeable, used their special talents in adulthood and went on to lead successful careers in the arts and sciences, one becoming a professor of astronomy to the extent of solving an error in the work of Sir Isaac Newton that he had originally noticed as a student. However, Asperger claimed that autistic traits were more often a disorder than a benefit for the majority of those who had them, and that those who were most severely impaired had little if any social worth, and were liable to become socially isolated because of their narrow interests.

Some years after his death, it was suggested that before and during the Second World War he had close links with the Nazi party and their death programmes aimed at killing off disabled children during the Second World War. However, no conclusive evidence that he had directly participated in any Nazi medical crimes was found, and two psychologists argued that far from being part of the ruling party's evil schemes, he attempted to protect children from being sent to concentration camps.

**Lorna Wing** (1928-2014), an English psychiatrist, initially trained as a doctor, specialising in psychiatry. Noted for her studies of childhood developmental disorders, she became involved in researching the subject in 1959 after she and her husband John realised that their daughter Susie, then aged three, was autistic, at a time when autism was thought to affect around five in 10,000 children. Susie had alarmed her parents because of her lack of communication and social interaction skills, lack of pretend play and repetitive behaviour. Neither parent, despite their medical training, had learned to recognise what they were seeing, and only when John attended a lecture by the child psychiatrist Mildred Creak did they recognise the problem. Lorna had already established a reputation for her electrophysiological studies of various types of mental illness, but she then abandoned them and devoted the rest of her career to studying and working on autism instead.

She was partly responsible for founding the National Autistic Society in Britain in 1962 and the Centre for Social and Communication Disorders in 1991. Her books and academic papers included *Asperger's syndrome: a Clinical Account* (1981), a paper which described thirty-four cases of children and adults with autism from five to thirty-five years, whose profiles of abilities did not easily match the diagnostic criteria for autism then in current usage by academics and clinicians, and which brought the terms Asperger syndrome and autistic spectrum disorder into common usage. A study of children in south London she undertook in 1979 revealed that all of those with social impairments had repetitive stereotyped behaviour, and most had an absence or abnormalities of language and symbolic activities, with a marked tendency for these problems to occur together.

# Autistic people in fact
# and fiction

We need to exercise great caution in suggesting that certain long-dead people were on the spectrum. Glen Elliott, a psychiatrist at the University of California at San Francisco, is among those who acknowledges that any kind of behaviour can have various causes, and attempting a diagnosis on the basis of biographical information is extremely unreliable. It is like the old conspiracy theory idea; historical facts can be arranged and stood on their head to prove any scenario one wants to. Yet several notable individuals in the past displayed certain traits which suggest that they might have been diagnosed had they been alive today.

One of the most famous 'possibles' was Wolfgang Amadeus Mozart, the composer, who had a tendency to make repeated facial expressions and was said to be hyperactive, rarely sitting still, constantly moving his hands and feet. He had very sensitive hearing, and loud sounds made him feel physically sick, was often unintentionally rude to people and suffered from regular mood changes.

A few members of British royalty were thought to have been affected. Albert, Prince Consort, was a solitary, introverted child who as an adult disliked parties, tended to fall asleep early, much to the irritation of Queen Victoria during their first years together. He hated trying to make small-talk, took everything very seriously, had little sense of humour, and would far rather converse at length on artistic or scientific interests with all the erudition or pedantry of a university professor. An inveterate workaholic who pushed himself to the limits and admitted he did not 'cling to life', he died at forty-two, apparently from an illness which may have been typhoid fever, stomach cancer or possibly Crohn's disease, but overwork was a contributory factor. His eldest daughter Victoria, Princess Royal, later German Empress and mother of 'Kaiser Bill' of the First World War, idolised him and inherited several of these traits to a marked degree. Recent research suggests that she had inherited the royal condition of porphyria, the most famous sufferer having been 'mad' King George III, but the possibility that she might have been on the spectrum cannot be ruled out.

Albert's great-grandson Prince John, the youngest son of King George V and Queen Mary, and 'The Lost Prince' of Stephen Poliakoff's television biopic, was another and even more likely case. Although full details were never fully made public, he was thought to have been diagnosed with epilepsy at the age of four, had learning difficulties and an inordinate fascination with repetitive routines in his day-to-day life. His epileptic seizures became more marked, and after a particularly severe one at the age of thirteen, he died in his sleep. His eldest brother, who was later briefly King Edward VIII and subsequently Duke of Windsor, wrote in his memoirs that his mother had very little understanding of a child's mind – as is often the case of autistic parents. One characteristic does not define somebody with ASD, but the possibility exists. To this list might be added Albert Victor, Duke of Clarence, eldest son of the future King Edward VII, and the man who would have become King but for his early death at the age of twenty-eight from influenza. As a child he had severe learning difficulties, and in youth was noted for being slow and lethargic. Conspiracy theorists have suggested on slender evidence that he may have been 'Jack the Ripper', responsible for a series of unsolved murders of prostitutes in the east end of London in 1888.

Andy Warhol, the artist, had an obsession with his love of repetition, such as the soup cans in his art, are thought to have been a manifestation of autism. John Peel, disc jockey and radio presenter, felt distinctly uncomfortable, even in later life, with socialising at parties. When his wife invited people around for the evening, he would spend an inordinate amount of time making cups of coffee or doing the washing up while everybody else partied happily in the next room.[14] There is a fine line between autism and extreme shyness or inability to communicate. Peel would doubtless have been in his element had guests wished to pick his brains on the finer points of the discography of one of his favourite groups. The list of present-day celebrities believed by some to be on the spectrum, and who have undergone what almost amounts to online diagnosis by fans, is almost endless – singer-songwriter Bob Dylan, actor and director Woody

Allen, Michael Palin of the *Monty Python* team, singer Michael Jackson, and former Kinks drummer Mick Avory, to name but a few.

Others who might have qualified for a diagnosis in the eyes of some include three of the greatest scientists of the last four centuries. According to autism expert Simon Baron-Cohen, of Cambridge University, and mathematician Ioan James of Oxford University, Sir Isaac Newton and Albert Einstein might both have shown signs of Asperger syndrome. Although he acknowledges that a definite diagnosis cannot be made for people long since dead, Baron-Cohen uses it as an example of how some affected people can become high achievers, while others feel positively disadvantaged. He assessed their personality traits of Newton and Einstein in terms of three key symptoms of Asperger syndrome: obsessive interests, difficulty in social relationships, and problems in communicating.

Newton was known for rarely speaking to others, and he often became so engrossed in his work that he forgot to eat regular meals. A lecturer on mathematics and science, and if nobody arrived to listen to his talks he gave them to an empty room. He was notoriously difficult to his very few friends. At the age of fifty he had a nervous breakdown, apparently caused by depression and paranoia. He fell out with most of the people with whom he had previously been on excellent terms, sending them fierce letters in which he accused them of various personal wrongdoings. After his death the writer Voltaire said that he 'was never sensible to any passion, was not subject to the common frailties of mankind, nor had any commerce with women —

a circumstance which was assured me by the physician and surgeon who attended him in his last moments'.

Einstein was a loner, especially as a child, and did not talk until he was three years old. Once he started, he was known for repeating the same sentences obsessively until about seven years of age, and although exceptionally intelligent – as his future career demonstrated beyond doubt - when at school had learning difficulties. Although he made several close friends, he experienced difficulties with social interaction. Unlike Newton, a lifelong bachelor, he married and became the father of three children, he could not stand letting the latter touch him. Like Newton, he was indifferent to such matters as issues of hygiene, regular mealtimes, and never seemed to be at all fussy about what he was eating.

The third was Charles Darwin. According to Professor Michael Fitzgerald of Trinity College, Dublin, the same genes that produce autism and Asperger syndrome also result in great creativity and originality. In Darwin's case they gave him the capacity to hyperfocus, an exceptional ability to see detail that was missed by others, endless energy for a lifetime dedication to a narrow task, and the independence of mind so critical to original research. A solitary child who devoted much time to collecting insects and shells, as a university student he became obsessed with chemistry and gadgets. In adult life he showed emotional immaturity and fear of intimacy, and although he became a devoted husband and father he avoided socialising as much as possible, happier when taking long walks on his own along the same daily route. The many letters that he wrote contained very little social chat.

Let us take the Newton, the Einstein, possibly even the Darwin, of the new millennium, Bill Gates of Microsoft, who is said to have Asperger syndrome. Those who have watched him speak have observed a wooden expression and a flat, monotone delivery. There is evidently a connection between scientific brilliance and the spectrum, as there seemingly is between Microsoft Corporation, apparently full of engineers and computer geeks with Asperger syndrome. Santa Clara County, the home of Microsoft Inc., reportedly has the highest rates of autism in the United States, 1:150, or one child in every 150. Children with it naturally gravitate towards careers such as engineering and computer science, and parents with it are more likely to have a child with an autistic spectrum disorder, adding to the hereditary factor. A retired NASA (National Aeronautics and Space Administration) space scientist once estimated that half his fellow engineers were probably on the spectrum. So perhaps was Steve Jobs of Apple Inc., who was known for little quirks as his obsession with perfection, his unorthodox ways of thinking, and his general lack of empathy when dealing with others.

On the subject of twentieth-century geniuses, Barbara McClintock, the scientist renowned for her pioneering study of chromosomes, had an extreme fixation on her work and the ability to focus for long periods of time, as well as being notoriously particular about what clothes she would and would not wear. For years she was a recluse who went to great lengths to avoid attention. A fellow scientist and her colleagues once paid her a visit in her laboratory, but she sent them away after half an hour because she thought they were being arrogant. One of them remarked as they left that she was either crazy or a genius'. She almost refused the 1983 Nobel Prize in Physiology or Medicine that she was awarded for her excellent and groundbreaking work. During her ninety years she never married, but in later years she evidently came to terms to some extent with her lack of social skills and led a more public life during which she accepted various honorary doctorates and awards, and gave talks on her research for the benefit of junior scientists.

Vincent van Gogh, the artist, had an unhappy early life and regularly gave evidence of behavioural problems, severe social impairment and problem at school. As an adult he found it almost impossible to interact with others, a loner and an outsider who inadvertently alienated people and had significant non-verbal behaviour problems. He was regarded as an eccentric and a workaholic who read books incessantly, narrowly focused on his art, responsible for a staggeringly prolific output of completed pictures during his last few months, often dressed in rags, had strange dietary habits, was not a fluent speaker, had severe mood swings, and less than two years after indulging in an astonishing act of self-harming by cutting off part of his ear, ended up by taking his own life.

One of his contemporaries was Henri ('Douanier') Rousseau, renowned as the most famous of the *naif* or 'primitive' artists. He showed several signs of being on the spectrum in his work and also in real life. His portraits of children and adults, and landscapes of Parisian suburbs, are often strangely childlike and lacking in perspective, and were ridiculed by critics. It was in his remarkable canvases of tropical jungles that he really fulfilled his potential, above all his gift for colour and his skills as a designer. As a personality he was simple and sometimes an easy prey to those who wished to take advantage of him, such as the occasion when thanks to the behaviour of a confidence trickster he found himself the unwitting innocent party in a case of minor fraud. Having outlived both his wives and most of his children, in his last years he became obsessed with a widow who refused to have anything to do with him, and neglected an infection in his leg that became gangrenous and proved fatal.

Going back to the Renaissance, Leonardo da Vinci, Italian Renaissance polymath, it is said, 'saw the world through a different prism than most of us'. With his brilliant, inventive mind, it was perhaps hardly surprising that his behaviour suggested Attention Deficit Disorder, hyperactivity and restlessness, and this his own letters and journals were single-minded, obsessive, and seemingly lacking in social grace or understanding. Michelangelo, a near-contemporary in a similar field, had similar characteristics. According to contemporary notes, letters and observations by others, he had an obsessive interest in his work, a sudden fiery temper, strict routines, and poor social skills.

In the literary world, two of the most noted nineteenth-century writers for children were thought to be on the spectrum. Hans Christian

Anderson, well-known for his fairy tales, is one case in point. There is a theory that most of those who insist that he was are autistic themselves, and can thus relate to him on a personal level. He left a diary that described at some length his frequent episodes of of unrequited love for those who were unattainable, said to be a common personal experience of those on the spectrum. Another often cited factor is the regularly recurring theme of outcast characters in his stories, with most of them failing to achieve the happy ending they seek so hard.

Lewis Carroll, the university professor, mathematical genius and self-proclaimed inventor who turned to writing fantasy in such titles as author of *Alice's Adventures in Wonderland*, had an obsession for the company of young girls. Some have seized on this as evidence of an unhealthy obsession if not an argument that he was a paedophile. Others suggest that he was autistic, with poor social and communication skills, exacerbated by a severe stammer, and thus found interacting with children much easier.

Emily Dickinson, the nineteenth-century poet, was a lifelong recluse who like Carroll much preferred the company of children to that of adults. Her other quirks included wearing white clothing almost exclusively, and a fascination with scented flowers.[15] While it was partly her epileptic condition that led her to shun human company so much, but as some medical professionals have stated, there is a strong connection between epilepsy and autism.

Turning to two early twentieth-century writers, firstly there is James Joyce. His titles such as the lengthy *Ulysses,* the semi-autobiographical *Portrait of the Artist as a Young Man,* and *Finnegan's Wake,* are generally categorised as brilliant yet very heavy going. He once said that the demand he made of his readers was that they should devote their whole life to reading his work, not a remark calculated to make friends and influence people. Some claim that such an approach to his work was either thoroughly eccentric or else characteristic of a wish to distance himself from society, in itself a sign of autism. Always very intelligent from his young days, he suffered from various phobias, and found it hard to make and keep friends.

Secondly, the poet William Butler Yeats had a difficult time at school where he was bullied for his lack of interest and awkward social behaviour. Later in life, she spent years pining for the always out-of-reach Maud Gonne, who showed no interest in him.

From the world of twentieth-century popular music, Michael Jackson, Syd Barrett of Pink Floyd and singer-songwriter Nick Drake are thought to have been on the spectrum. The former had savant-like talents, and wrote some of the most popular songs of the era by imitating the sounds of musical instruments with his vocal chords although evidence suggests that he never really mastered any of them, perhaps because he never needed to, engaged in repetitive rituals, which helped him to hone his dance moves to perfection, and was so poor at making eye contact that he conducted most of his interviews wearing sunglasses. Both the latter were also highly creative and imaginative personalities with severe communication difficulties, very withdrawn at social gatherings, and hated performing onstage. Consumption of recreational drugs probably increased their paranoia, resulting in Barrett leading an unfulfilled life as a recluse for nearly forty years between being fired by his bandmates and his death, and Drake dying from a possibly intentional drug overdose at the age of twenty-six, but self-indulgence may have done no more than exacerbate the conditions that were already there.

Bobby Fischer, the chess grandmaster and World Chess Champion, reportedly had Asperger's as well as paranoid schizophrenia and Obsessive Compulsive Disorder. He was known to be extremely intense, for not relating well to others because of his lack of friendships and poor social abilities, for his extreme focus on chess, and his problems with coping in an unstructured environment.

Several living people have spoken about their experiences of being on the spectrum, or of having close relations who had been affected. They – and many others - are the living proof that being autistic is no barrier to having a successful career, but all readily acknowledge that a diagnosis can help make life, or an ongoing stressful situation, much easier for them.

Elfriede Jelinek, playwright, novelist, and winner of the Novel Prize for Literature in 2004, was a hyperactive small child who would run from room to room for hours on end. This unnerved her mother, who took her to Hans Asperger as a patient. He diagnosed her 'as prey to an excitement which had yet to find a suitable outlet'. With some bitterness, she never forgot that 'instead of sending me out to play in the company of kids my age, my mother sent me into the company of severe neurotics and psychopaths'. After completing her school education she went to study Art History and Theatre at Vienna University, but had to leave her course early because of a severe anxiety disorder. Kept in isolation at her parents' house for a year, she began to write as a form of therapy.

Paddy Considine, actor, was diagnosed with Asperger syndrome at the age of thirty-six. At eighteen he went to the doctor and tried to explain that he felt a sense of detachment between himself and the rest of the world. After being offered 'the usual antidepressant therapy' and being threatened with hospitalisation, he went to college and university, armed with the belief that if he worked hard enough and achieved some success, his problems would just leave him. It did not work, 'because Asperger's is not something you just get over or grow out of.' The 'debilitating sense of detachment' from both the people around him and his surroundings, and struggles on a practical level with certain noises, bright lights, and even wallpaper and fabrics like brightly coloured, geometrically striped carpets made life difficult. His wife was convinced he had several of the symptoms of Asperger's, and could see that he was getting to a real low point in his life where the strategies he was using to cope were hurting him, and insisted that he went to see a specialist. For a few weeks after the diagnosis he was wandering around thinking, 'Who the hell am I?' Nevertheless it helped him in allowing him to make sense of so much he never understood before, and it was 'allowing me to move forward with my life.'[16]

Mary Temple Grandin, equally well-known as a professor of Animal Science, consultant to the livestock industry on animal behaviour, and spokesperson on autism, did not begin talking until she was three and a half years old. She was never formally diagnosed as being on the spectrum in childhood or in youth, and her only formal diagnosis was of 'brain damage' at the age of two, corroborated some sixty years later by cerebral imaging. Her schooldays were troubled, especially by students who would taunt her by calling her 'tape recorder' because of her habit of repetitive speech, and she was expelled at the age of fourteen for throwing a book at a schoolmate who had teased her. During her adolescence, her mother found a checklist on autism, and on studying it concluded that her symptoms were best explained by autism, although a formal diagnosis consistent with being on the spectrum was made only when she was in her forties.

Gary Numan, singer and musician, was a loner as a child, and always felt happiest at home playing with his toy rockets and aeroplanes. When he 'started causing trouble' in his third year at grammar school, his parents sent him to a child psychologist, who suggested he might have Asperger's, although he never had a formal diagnosis. Some people seem concerned about it, he says, but he has turned it to advantage and always seen it as a positive thing. While admitting that he may be somewhat awkward socially, he considers it a small price to pay for the advantages. Being obsessive can be a benefit in certain careers, and a vital and useful trait for people in the music business. He readily admits to being 'driven and highly focused' on things in which he is interested in, like his musical career. 'My emotional differences mean that I am able to shrug of criticism with barely a second thought and nothing, absolutely nothing, swerves me from my intended goal.' Although he is not good at eye contact, he finds ways of dealing with that, and as he finds casual conversations stressful, he avoids them whenever possible. As his wife has a similarly affected brother, she is familiar with and understands the differences; 'she tolerates some, and enjoys others, because many of those differences are actually beneficial. I wouldn't change me.'[17]

Jerry Seinfeld, the comedian, has also never been officially diagnosed by a medical professional. He has said in interviews that he believes himself to be on the autism spectrum, defending his self-diagnosis by citing various social challenges that he has experienced since childhood, and also a tendency to think literally. Some authorities in the autism community disagree, and consider that his self-diagnosis has only served to make light of actual issues.

Among other famous names, it is perhaps only appropriate as well as significant that one of the people who has publicly revealed most about his life on the spectrum is a well-known British broadcaster. Chris Packham, the wildlife television presenter, was diagnosed with Asperger syndrome in 2005 at the age of forty-four. In his memoirs, *Fingers in the Sparkle Jar*, published eleven years later, and a BBC television documentary, *Aspergers and Me*, first shown a year after that, he wrote and spoke in detail of his introverted early years, of a love affair with natural history and his joy in raising a young kestrel, and of contemplating suicide after the death of one of his dogs, but was dissuaded from such a drastic step as he could not let the other dogs down. From a young age he was in his own words 'an intense observer' who could see things in nature which others could not. His mother used to tease him about his ability to recognise individual caterpillars, as to her they all looked the same. At school he was rejected by his peers, picked on and felt totally excluded. When he went to university he still had this feeling of being 'different' yet not knowing why, and had to develop his own ways of dealing with it. His strategy was not to interact with or even speak to anyone unless absolutely necessary, but just persevere with his academic work and focus on getting good grades at the end of his course.

In the 1970s his parents and their peers were completely unfamiliar with autism 'and there was no real ability to diagnose or understand it. Now there is.' Only when he was in his early forties did he recognise that he needed to seek professional help. After his diagnosis, he expressed concern that accessing assistance at that level was not open to everybody who needed it, partly because of significant funding issues and partly the lack of access to qualified staff. He felt empowered to speak publicly about mental health issues, bringing them into the forum of discussion.

'We need to generate more awareness of the fact that peoples' families and friends are not necessarily the best people to help,' he said. 'They may want to help, but they just may not be able to. Therefore we need access to people who can, and we have to make sure that's freely available and not just for people who can afford it and that it's accessible at the right time.'[18]

In the documentary, he referred to having been with his partner for ten years, though they both have their own space. Speaking about their relationship, he acknowledged that he was very lucky to have found someone who was prepared to put up with the constant social failings caused by his Aspergers, while she spoke of a 'lifetime guarantee' that she would never be bored with or by him. After ten years, she was still 'fascinated by his mind'. From the days when he first appeared as a fresh-faced adult on children's television talking about wildlife, but when his diagnosis was still some years in the future, he realised that the indefinable factor that made him 'different' and enabled him to use his encyclopaedic knowledge of the animal world, and find his level in a world where he was really at home. While he admits that he has an enormous job managing his condition and finds it quite draining at times, he could not do the job he loves if he did not have Aspergers. If he was offered a cure, he would not hesitate in refusing it.

Dan Aykroyd, actor and comedian, was diagnosed with Tourette syndrome at the age of twelve, with physical tics, nervousness, obsessive compulsive disorder and a tendency to make grunting noises, but the symptoms had eased with therapy two years later. In his early thirties his wife persuaded him to see a doctor because they were convinced he was autistic. About twenty years later, he said that Asperger's had been diagnosed but he could 'manage it'. A couple of years after that he remarked in another interview that it was never formally confirmed but was 'sort of a self-diagnosis' based on several of his characteristics.

Susan Boyle, the singer who became famous after appearing on television's *Britain's Got Talent*, was misdiagnosed with brain damage after complications at birth, was bullied when she was a child and suffered for years from depression and mood swings. Convinced that she had a serious illness and 'couldn't function properly', at the age of fifty-one she consulted a specialist and was diagnosed with Asperger syndrome. 'It will not make any difference to my life,' she said in an interview. 'It's just a condition that I have to live with and work through. Now I have a clearer understanding of what's wrong and I feel relieved and a bit more relaxed about myself.'[19]

Helena Bonham-Carter, actress and former wife of producer-director Tim Burton, once described how they were watching a documentary about autism together and he told her that that was how he felt as a child. He has not been formally diagnosed although he has several of the characteristics, including a lack of social skills despite being highly intelligent, a tendency to hyperfocus on specific interests, and a love of dressing in black clothes as he does not like to spend (or waste) too much time selecting matching colours. He has a pronounced sense of humour and imagination, thus giving the lie to the generalisation that such people lack both these qualities.

# Autistic people in music,
# film and television

Many song lyrics are notoriously open to interpretation in more than one way, but Paul Simon's *The Sound of Silence*, as recorded by him and Art Garfunkel in 1965, might be seen in part as a song about autism on a wide scale. Garfunkel has said that it is basically about 'the inability of people to communicate with each other, not particularly internationally but especially emotionally, so what you see around you are people unable to love each other'. Another of Simon's songs which appeared on the same album, *I am a Rock*, is written in the first person from the point of view of someone reveling in isolation – 'I've built walls, a fortress deep and mighty, that none may penetrate', and the last verse finishes with 'And a rock feels no pain, and an island never cries'. It could be taken as a *cri de coeur* from somebody who is determined to isolate him/herself from human company for fear of getting hurt, or equally from that of someone who is autistic.[20]

The American road comedy-drama *Rain Man* tells the story of young hustler Charlie Babbitt (Tom Cruise) and his discovery that his estranged father has recently died, leaving his estate to his older son Raymond (Dustin Hoffman), of whose existence Charlie has never been aware until then. Raymond, who lives in a mental home, is autistic, has very good recall of certain events, only feels comfortable with strict routines, such as being in bed by 11.00 p.m. every night without fail, and shows little emotional expression except when distressed. When Charlie meets him, he discovers that he also has an inbuilt ability to count hundreds of objects at the same time.

Some darker popular situation comedies and dramas feature leading characters who could be said to be on the spectrum. Mr Bean (Rowan Atkinson), 'a child in a grown man's body', of the eponymous series, is a case in point. So is Basil Fawlty (John Cleese) of *Fawlty Towers*, the appallingly rude, snobbish, sarcastic, easily panicked and stressed hotelier who seems to find safety in keeping doggedly to the same routines as much as possible, is a case in point. So is another character later played by Cleese, Brian Stimpson, the unbelievably organised comprehensive school headmaster of *Clockwise*, with his fanatical insistence of doing everything and seeing everyone at a precise time. He goes completely to pieces on his big day at a prestigious headmasters' conference when he accidentally gets on the wrong train, leading to several hours of almost surreal hilarious yet nightmarish mishaps, in which the poignant sight of a well-meaning individual, the victim of his own obsessions, is never completely submerged. By tragic coincidence, a real life Brian Stimpson, an unemployed single man of forty from Gravesend, made several suicide attempts before dousing himself in petrol and setting light to himself in 2013, dying from his injuries three days later. At an inquest, the coroner's evidence suggested that he was 'nervous around people he did not know', and although undiagnosed he was probably autistic.

Martin Bryce (Richard Briers), the central character of the sitcom *Ever Decreasing Circles*, is another instance of a semi-comic, semi-serious character with a similar problem. An obsessive suburban busybody, he is devoted to organising committees in the local community, doing everything the same way, insisting that the receiver on the landline telephone (a few years before the advent of cordless and mobile phones) is always replaced the same way, earnestly making a written note of every little trivial detail down when the mildly exasperated local policeman is briefing him about his duties and responsibilities in the local Neighbourhood Watch scheme, and sitting at exactly the same table in the pub. In the process he frequently exasperates his long-suffering wife Ann (Penelope Wilton) who however realises she cannot change him, and amuses his 'come-on-life-amuse-me' neighbour Paul Ryman (Peter Egan), who seems to be able to do everything so effortlessly, knows all the right people, and cannot resist the temptation to make fun of him while regularly performing acts of kindness for them both. While the last series was coming to an end, a girl with whom I was going out for a short time once asked me whether I wouldn't rather be more like Paul than Martin. It occurred to me while I was watching some of the repeat runs about thirty years later that she might in some vague way have put her finger on the problem.

Dr Martin Ellingham (Martin Clunes) of *Doc Martin* is another. As the local doctor in a close-knit Cornish village community, he lacks social skills, empathy and the right bedside manner, appears hot-tempered, resents wasting valuable time with small talk, always dresses formally in a business suit and tie, regardless of the weather or the occasion, and never takes off his jacket, even when delivering babies. He and his wife have a son, but his apparent inability to show her any affection places their marriage under strain.

Finally, Mark Haddon's novel *The Curious Incident of the Dog in the Night-time* (or *the curious incident of the dog in the night-time* as the title appears within the book) has an autistic hero – though admittedly an adolescent, not an adult. I am not referring to the canine, but to Christopher, the narrator. (The lower-case letters alluded to are relevant). An intelligent lad aged fifteen who turns detective after the animal next door is killed, he is clearly on the spectrum. Very knowledgeable about mathematics but not about human beings, he displays many of the aspects of the condition such as having an aversion to the colours yellow and brown, levels of noise, and being touched.

# The adult problem of autism

A widespread belief that autism was seen largely, and inaccurately, as something associated with children was confirmed in 2013 when the National Autistic Society (NAS) Scotland warned of an 'invisible generation' of older people on the spectrum in Scotland whose condition was often misunderstood and misdiagnosed. One in five people with autism, it concluded, or more than 11,600 of 58,000 north of the Scottish border, was thought to be over the age of sixty. The Society called for action to ensure the needs of elderly people with autism were fully understood and met, and urged the Scottish government to act on its concerns in implements a ten-year Autism Strategy for Scotland, addressing the entire autism spectrum and the whole lifespan of people living with the condition in Scotland, and rolling out over £13,000,000 in funding to support those affected.

A recent survey of adults with autism had revealed that more than a third had been waiting three years or more to access a diagnosis. Moreover, with little existing research into how the condition would develop in older age, there was also some doubt over the form effective support would take in the long term for those with autism. It said it had received anecdotal evidence that clinicians working in age-related specialisms tended to have a poor understanding of the disability and limited professional understanding on how health issues such as dementia might affect adults with autism.

Robert MacBean, policy and campaigns officer for NAS Scotland, said that tremendous progress had been made in recent years in changing attitudes towards autism and increasing understanding of the lifelong, disabling condition that touched the lives of those who were affected. Despite this, not enough attention was paid to older people with autism in all communities who still needed support and care, too many of whom were missing out on diagnosis entirely and too many were still waiting for their needs to be assessed. Moreover it was uncertain what support they would receive as they got older.

One such person was retired joiner David Silvester, who was diagnosed with Asperger syndrome two years previously, at the age of sixty-five. His condition had been misdiagnosed as bipolar disorder and schizophrenia when he was in his twenties, around forty years previously. His diagnosis, he said, came as a huge relief. For most of his adult life he had questioned what was really wrong with him. 'The diagnosis finally explained my life, who I am and took away a lot of the negative feelings I'd projected onto myself. When I was very young, research into Asperger syndrome was also in its infancy. But I'd known from an early age that I was "different". If the adults around me had known what to look for, they would have seen classic Asperger traits. On the outside I appeared articulate and functioning well. But inside I was struggling.'

He was still struggling afterwards. After his diagnosis, he thought a world of support services in his area would open up to him, and it was a major disappointment when he found otherwise. Once his local council began developing its Autism Strategy, he became involved in educating people about autism and encouraging decision-makers to put in place effective support. He said it would be tremendous if the public could see that older people with autism were not 'weird' or 'odd'. 'We just see the world in a different way. We need the right support at the right time, but we also have skills, talents and abilities.'[21]

Young adults are equally deserving of the right support. With their attention to detail, people on the spectrum have very strong potential as students – as long as they can overcome the hurdle of entering life in the campus in the first place. This was the experience of Hannah Khan, a high-achieving first year-student on a computer science degree course at the University of Bath, who was diagnosed at the age of fourteen. At first she admitted she did not know what it meant; 'all you've got on the internet are things saying how negative it is, how I'll have trouble for the rest of my life.' She was hypersensitive to noise and touch. 'If someone tapped me on the shoulder it would feel like a burning sensation. It's really unpleasant and horrible. If there were loud and sudden noises, I'd be anxious and startled. It sends waves of panic through me. People look at you in a confused way - they don't understand the sensitivity. They don't understand why I jump away and freak out.'[1]

Although later told she should not be in mainstream education, she was determined to succeed. In her view many autistic people are scared of university, and 'get pushed down a route they don't want to go down.' Being autistic at university can be 'very tough', but many people on the spectrum were not even given the chance, and instead consigned to low achievement and low expectations. According to the university, fewer than one in six autistic adults are in full-time jobs, and even those who have work can be stuck in roles far below their ability. Having 'been to a lot of things where you get pushed around as the "autistic person"',' she was very hesitant about applying to university until a summer school convinced her that it was well within her reach. Her communication with other people was 'very complicated …I can't talk in a group setting and sometimes it just falls apart a bit. The words are in my head and the language is there, but there's a kind of break between that I can't seem to cross … In freshers' week, when everyone is out getting to know each other, you're sat there thinking "'I don't know if I can talk to all these people".' Navigating social situations could be uncomfortable. She often felt 'disconnected' and missed out on social activities, when other students assumed she would not want to come along. For her, saying hello to people and getting to know them meant a huge emotional effort, that was not always recognised and left her at the risk of being silently 'hurt'. The experience convinced her that universities needed to have specialised, psychiatric and psychological support for autistic students with many different and complex needs, and she questioned whether conventional counselling or mentoring was adequate.[1]

# Can autism and Asperger syndrome be cured?

Yes, they can.

No, they cannot. Do they need to be?

As with so many things, ask different people and get different answers. I recently came across a couple of threads on an online forum which sparked off a lively and for the most part good-tempered debate on the subject. If you are on the spectrum, as I have already said, as you have to live with it you can manage it to a certain extent, particularly with moral support in the family and workplace, you can adapt, and you can learn to overcome the problems. Personally, I believe that this is not the same thing as a cure. Some maintain that high functioning autism, not Kanner syndrome, can be cured, as it is a communication disorder, not a different brain. They also insist that those on the spectrum can learn non-verbal communication, and no less importantly, how to deal with change. It does not however help to address the issue when society, perhaps out of political correctness and recognition of equal opportunities for all, is seen to have a principle of 'celebrating diversity' in preference instead of teaching the basic skills for human interaction.

Most people agree that living successfully with the condition and meeting the challenges halfway stops short of cure. Simon Baron-Cohen maintains that for those on the spectrum, it is possible to adapt their personality to the outside world when needed, 'but one's personality ultimately is who you are, and aspects of the core (such as excellent attention to detail and sensory hyper-sensitivity) do not fundamentally change across one's life.' For some people, social skills can be acquired, and thus improve to varying degrees, with age and experience. Some hold that his view on autism is open to question as he effectively blames the brain for creating 'one size fits all' strategies for explanations of the condition, although in this case at least his view seems perfectly plausible. People in jobs or those who are self-employed may be lacking in social skills but have that all-important eye for detail, such as proof readers or excellent specialist knowledge in their chosen field – as good an example of adaptation in the outside world as any.

One contributor to the threads, who had Asperger syndrome, said he or she could testify that it is possible for like-minded people to push boundaries, challenge themselves, adapt to the best of their ability - and achieve success in life. This did not alter the fact that the same anxieties persisted; people merely learn to manage them better, but this comes at a cost. Adaptation 'is exhausting', often results in individuals finding it mentally demanding being 'normal', getting tired at the end of the day and, like Greta Garbo, just wanting to be alone. Another claimed that he or she knew two prominent (and unnamed) psychologists who believed that autism could be cured. The same contributor claimed to know someone who had not only cured themselves of Asperger's but had also read a book by someone else who cured themselves, and maintained that there was is no difference between a non-autistic and an autistic brain.

It has been argued, and convincingly to an extent, that those with high-functioning autism find it easier to interact more easily with others and can cope more easily with changes to their routines, either through sheer determination or by being taught. Yet when all is said and done it does not amount to a cure, as the person still sees the world differently; it is a major part of who they are, so there is probably no need for a cure. I say 'probably', as fears have been voiced that if an officially recognised 'cure' should come, for potential members of the workforce there might not be a choice, should legislation be introduced – in Britain, America or anywhere else – for people who have been diagnosed to undergo treatment or discriminated against through coercion in that they would not be hired otherwise. In other words, choosing not to take the cure could be seen as proof of wilfulness, lack of competence or even mental disorder.

Some people, notably Jim Sinclair, autism rights movement activist and co-founder of Autism Network International, are standard bearers for those who do not want autism cured. In a significant article which has provoked a wide-ranging debate since publication over twenty years ago, he argued that autism is a way of being. 'It is *pervasive*; it colours every experience, every sensation, perception, thought, emotion, and encounter, every aspect of existence. It is not possible to separate the autism from the person--and if it were possible, the person you'd have left would not be the same person you started with.' His arguments have been taken as expression of accepting the status quo, to the extent of not wanting autism 'cured'. The ways that autistic people such as himself relate to everything and everyone else, he maintained, are different.

> Push for the things your expectations tell you are normal, and you'll find frustration, disappointment, resentment, maybe even rage and hatred. Approach respectfully, without preconceptions, and with openness to learning new things, and you'll find a world you could never have imagined. Yes, that takes more work than relating to a non-autistic person. But it *can* be done - unless non-autistic people are far more limited than we are in their capacity to relate. We spend our entire lives doing it. Each of us who does learn to talk to you, each of us who manages to function at all in your society, each of us who manages to reach out and make a connection with you, is operating in alien territory, making contact with alien beings. We spend our entire lives doing this. And then you tell us that we can't relate.[22]

This approach has been backed up by the school of thought that indicates there are physical brain differences between autistic and neuro-typical people - and that cannot be cured. To talk of cures, it has been said, is reminiscent of those people who say they can 'cure' homosexuality.

Occasionally autistic people (or those thought to be on the spectrum) reach the stage where they no longer meet the criteria for a diagnosis. This may be because they have initially been misdiagnosed, or children who mature out of certain forms of autism and 'lose their diagnosis', but this rarely applies to adults. There is also the possibility – but little more than a possibility - that successful treatment can, in some instances, produce outcomes that no longer meet the criteria for an autism diagnosis.

Interventions, in the form of treatments and therapies, have been designed to improve the quality of life for adults with autism. There is no one-size fits all solution, and the most effective interventions have been devised to meet the unique characteristics of each individual. NICE (National Institute for Health and Care Excellence) provides national guidance and advice to improve health and social care, and has published several documents on the care of adults on the autism spectrum.

Other interventions include AAT (assistive and adaptive technology, or products, devices or equipment, whether acquired commercially, modified or customised, used to maintain, increase or improve the functional capabilities of individuals with disabilities; AAC, or any form of communication that people use if they are unable or unwilling to use standard forms of communication such as speech, including sign language and voice output communication aids; Behavioural and Developmental Interventions, designed to encourage appropriate behaviour that which is inappropriate, such as self-harm or aggression towards others, and to target the core deficits within the individual rather than his or her outward behaviours; such as ABA (applied behaviour analysis), CBT (cognitive behaviour therapy), functional communication training, positive behavioural support, self-management, and social skills groups. Others comprise Dietary Supplements, intended to be taken by mouth as a pill, capsule, tablet, or liquid; Special Diets, which involve eating more or less of specific foodstuffs; Vocational Interventions, activities designed to help people on the spectrum find, get and keep a job, or enable them to improve the workplace experience and enhance their careers; Medications intended for use in the medical diagnosis, cure, treatment, or prevention of disease, such as anticonvulsants, antidepressants such as fluoxetine, antipsychotics such as risperidone, cholinesterase Inhibitors such as donepezil, and stimulants such as methtylphenidate; Motor Sensory Interventions, any treatments and therapies which make use of or which aim to improve motor functioning, or movement of the whole body or parts of the body; Psychological interventions, which comprise a wide range of interventions based on how we think, feel, act and interact, individually and in groups, among them counselling, psychotherapy, cognitive and behavioural therapies; and Social care services, designed for assessing the needs of, and providing support to people on the autism spectrum in the community, normally provided by the local social services/social work department, by a social enterprise or not-for-profit organisation, or by a parent or carer. Finally there is Standard Health Care, or conventional medicine, to maintain the health and well-being of individuals with autism. This includes medication, occupational therapy, osteopathy, physiotherapy, psychology, psychotherapy, and speech and language therapy (speech pathology), and comprises a wide range of treatments and therapies accepted and used by the majority of health care professionals, among them occupational therapists, psychologists and speech and language therapists who often work together using a combination of behavioural, developmental, AAC and motor-sensory interventions.[23]

# Autism and addictions

A study by the Mental Health Foundation in 2006 found that 65% of alcoholics admitted to rehab suffered from social anxiety. Significantly, some of these were almost certainly undiagnosed autistic people.

At around the same time, a close examination of links between autism and alcohol abuse was carried out by Sarah Hendrickx and Matthew Tinsley, the former an expert on working in the autism field and the latter an autistic friend and recovering alcoholic, and their findings were published in 2008. Their research was hampered by the fact that many adults are undiagnosed, and alcohol can act as a successful coping strategy which hides autistic difficulties for many years before the alcohol becomes a problem in itself.

Tinsley was able to speak from experience, as the chief aspect of his autism which resulted in heavy alcohol consumption to cope was a near constant sense of anxiety. Being socially awkward, he discovered that alcohol made him a much more relaxed person. He was unaware of his autism at the time and it was only in retrospect that he could appreciate why it worked so well. Alcohol enabled him to function in the workplace and develop and maintain relationships, helped him to be less affected by sensory stressors, to manage his anxiety and to reduce the impact of his autism.

Sensory problems which he had such as loud noises and certain textured clothes being uncomfortable could always be numbed to an extent by drink. Being overwhelmed with information when being given instructions was also not a problem when drinking as he felt able to retain the information. Alcohol enabled him to do jobs where anxiety might have been crippling, involving working in an environment with constant contact with the public. Despite being technically drunk, he was very efficient at his jobs and coped well with them for seventeen years, until the situation became life–threatening with liver damage and potentially fatal consequences if he did not stop drinking.

The solution in his case was a residential CBT (Cognitive Behaviour Therapy) rehabilitation unit and a complete change of lifestyle, which allowed him to live alcohol-free for several years. His diagnosis gave him the knowledge to realise his own anxiety as an autistic person, and his need to reduce the demands upon him.[24]

Although I never became an alcoholic myself, I will admit that I too had times of heavy drinking for similar reasons before I knew I was on the spectrum. My paternal grandmother, who died in her early sixties many years before I was born, was an alcoholic and spent her last years in a nursing home. My father never spoke about her to us, but he had what I would call quite a relaxed attitude to alcohol consumption in the home or socially, as long as kept within reasonable bounds, never trying to preach about the evils of the bottle – which, in view of family history, some might consider he was entitled to do. My mother once alluded to a cousin or uncle on her side of the family who probably drank himself into an early grave. In my case, I think I was fortunate enough to realise when to stop before I ran the risk of damaging my liver.

It is hardly surprising that some autistic people are tempted to use alcohol as a way of warding off the anxiety which they suffer as a result of their condition, and those who are possibly undiagnosed cannot access support as the removal of the alcohol may in extreme cases make them incapable of leaving the house. More awareness of the potential of autism resulting in problem drinking is required within alcohol support services, with patients generally required to be 'dry' before receiving treatment, and there needs to be recognition of the signs as this type of client may have no autism diagnosis. The signs to look for that a person with an alcohol problem might also be autistic could be unusual eye-contact, special interests, their use of language with regard to unusual grammar and pedantic syntax.

Some people are more at risk of developing addiction to alcohol or drugs than others, perhaps due to hereditary factors or due to the environment of the individual. Those who feel alienated from other people and struggle with social interactions appear particularly prone to substance abuse, as alcohol or drugs can make people feel more sociable while making them less self-conscious, and those on the autistic spectrum may be at greater risk of addiction.

Self-knowledge of autism which can come as a result of an official diagnosis can be helpful to someone with a drink problem to be aware of their condition, and why they find life sometimes overwhelms them. Alcohol services may need to consider alternative approaches for treatment that meet the needs of the autistic cognitive profile which may be substantially different. Cognitive Behaviour Therapy adapted for use with autistic people can be extremely beneficial in helping to support the core anxiety which may be at the root of the need for alcohol.

Another study, carried out at Washington University School of Medicine, St Louis, published in 2014, concluded that young adults with autistic tendencies did not often engage in social or binge drinking, but if they drank, they were more likely than their peers to develop alcohol problems. The researchers did not study people with autism, but wanted to find out whether traits linked to the condition, such as social-interaction difficulties, communication challenges and a tendency to engage in repetitive behaviour, put people at risk for alcohol and other substance-use problems. It concluded that as drinking to intoxication was a social activity more likely to occur in a group, and as people with autistic traits could be be socially withdrawn, drinking with peers was less likely. However if they started drinking, even alone, they had a tendency to repeat that behaviour, which would put them at increased risk for alcohol dependence.

# Autism, stress, mental health, anxiety and depression

There is a distinct correlation between all four. For a long time prior to my diagnosis, I was sure that my problems were the result of stress, anxiety and depression. They have not been vanquished with a wave of the magic wand in my post-diagnostic existence, but significantly reduced. The research group Research Autism launched a campaign, Beating Stress in Autism in 2016, to address the effects of stress on autistic people and their families. It coincided with an article by Richard Mills, Research Director, which outlines how stress can affect autistic people, their families and the professionals who work with them. The sense of being under too much mental or emotional pressure turns into stress when you feel unable to cope, and helps us to distinguish between stress, usually a result of external forces and anxiety, which is more frequently found within the person and manifests in the form of worrying, and persistent thoughts. Too often the two are joined together and, although related, they are different and the approaches to manage them will need to reflect this. Stress is often described as a major barrier to a fulfilled life for autistic people and affects everyone, especially people on the autism spectrum at all stages of their lives.

Autistic people can be especially susceptible to high levels of unhealthy stress. Sometimes the reason may be unclear, related to underlying insecurity, uncertainty, or to sensory processing problems that might not be apparent, even to the person concerned. The results can be tiredness, irritability or lack of concentration, and the sensory profile of autism may be related to how well a person copes with stress and is a factor in depression. Research shows that autistic boys with a sensory seeking profile (low registration) are much more prone to developing severe depression. This suggests that assessment of the sensory profile is important, as is the adoption of methods or activities to address these particular needs.

In the case of adults, who may also be struggling with minor issues of short-term memory impairment, the issue can be more pronounced. A woman who was diagnosed with autism at the age of sixty-six, speaking about her experiences on the radio a few months later, said that from her experience, auditory processing of information and short-term memory were particularly difficult. She herself had been asked sometimes whether she had hearing difficulties, as she was sometimes slow to respond to questions and it took her a long time to process the information coming to her. The psychologist whom she saw as part of her diagnosis told her that she and others like her had to work at least twice as hard as 'ordinary people' to make sense of information, as they were slow to pick up meaning and detail as their brains were making an exceptional effort to make sense of what they are being told.[25]

Some key areas to explore include the phenomena known as 'meltdowns', 'shutdowns' and 'catatonia', which may all be manifestations of stress and be related to feelings of powerlessness or lack of control over stressor events. The build-up may go unnoticed until it is too late. These aspects are poorly understood, especially shutdown and catatonia, and further research is needed to understand them better.

The most common signs of stress include feeling anxious and irritable, having low self-esteem, racing thoughts, constant worry, having to go over things again and again in your head, losing your temper, appearing unreasonable, headaches, muscle tension, pain, dizziness and not finding enjoyment in things you have previously enjoyed. It is also known to cause a surge of hormones called stress hormones, which are designed to react to stressful situations known as the 'fight or flight' response. In most people, these usually return to normal levels once the stressful event has passed. Those who are autistic are more vulnerable as these hormones tend to remain in the body for longer, causing a residual level of stress, resulting in potentially harmful physical and psychological effects of too much stress over a prolonged period. They can lead to other problems, such as drinking too much alcohol or taking drugs to offset the effects. There may also be a tendency for autistic people to self-medicate if he or she is unable to access support or cannot easily identify the sources of stress. This may be exacerbated by a poor diet, as he or she may lose their appetite and not eat properly. It may lead to additional problems at work or with sleeping. In some instances, stress has been dealt with by overuse of antipsychotic medication to subdue behaviour. Non-speaking autistic people, unable to communicate stress or distress, can be particularly susceptible to this problem.

It is important to help people to identify the sources and mechanisms of stress and to develop coping strategies, or stress hygiene. These comprise regular exercise, learning how to relax, a structured timetable to allow for time management and to build in wind–down periods, and time spent in relaxation. In work with women, 'masking' of autism symptoms was described as a major source of stress, causing us to reflect on whether those interventions aimed at reducing those symptoms may be inherently stressful and bad for autistic people.

Autistic people are liable to experience high levels of stress in everyday life. Chronic stress reduces the ability to participate properly in academic, work, leisure, and social life and heightens the risk of physical ill-health. Subjective experience of stress, coping ability and sensory profiles are all huge contributors and should be assessed in conjunction with the assessment of autism.

The Research Autism initiative has recognised that it is stress and not autism that has become a major barrier in life for many people on the spectrum and this should receive the attention it merits from research, policy and practice. The solutions will be found through an alliance of autistic people, their families and the professional autism and research communities.

Approaches that enable the person to control or moderate their stress would seem particularly important.[26]

Depression is generally reckoned to be a period of low mood that, rather than lifting after a few days or perhaps even weeks, lasts longer and gets in the way of day-to-day functioning. It is generally accompanied by feelings of worthlessness, hopelessness, helplessness and low self-esteem, feeling tearful, guilt-ridden, irritable and intolerant of others, losing motivation and interest in things, finding it difficult to make decisions, not getting any enjoyment out of life, and thoughts of self-harm or even worse. It affects people in different ways and can cause a wide variety of symptoms ranging from lasting feelings of unhappiness and hopelessness, to losing interest in things they used to enjoy and feeling prone to tears. The physical symptoms include disturbed sleep, with finding it hard to fall asleep at night or waking up very early in the morning, leading to constant feelings of tiredness, loss of energy, appetite or sex drive, various aches and pains, moving or speaking more slowly than usual, and changes in appetite or weight.

Depression affects non-autistic people, probably at least 20% of the population at some point in their lives, but is more common in people on the spectrum. According to a study published in 2015 in California, adults with autism are three times more likely to have depression, and five times more likely to attempt suicide, than the general population. Almost half of the people who tried to take their lives had not been diagnosed with depression before their attempts, and people with high functioning autism, those who are verbal and do not have intellectual disability, are probably at higher risk of depression. Research suggests that its symptoms may hide behind some of the common features of autism, such as an emotionless expression or voice, sleep problems, and trouble concentrating. Rather than looking tired and sad, a depressed person with autism may have a tendency to appear irritable, agitated, or be liable to emotional outbursts.[27]

Many people with depression also have symptoms of anxiety or GAD (generalised anxiety disorder). It can cause a change in behaviour and the way people think and feel about things, resulting in restlessness, a sense of dread, feeling constantly 'on edge', difficulty concentrating, and irritability. People suffering from it may try to withdraw from seeing family and friends in order to avoid feelings of worry and dread. They may find going to work difficult and stressful, maybe even impossible, about themselves and increase their lack of self-esteem. Physical symptoms include dizziness, tiredness, palpitations or a noticeably strong, fast or irregular heartbeat, muscle aches and tension, trembling or shaking, dry mouth, excessive sweating, shortness of breath, stomachache, headache, nausea, and insomnia.[28]

People with any of these disorders can experience a range of symptoms which vary from person to person in their combination, and can be mild or severe. It is often hard for depressed people on the autism spectrum to seek help as they might find change daunting and anxiety-provoking, feel worried that they will be blamed, or feel unsure about how to describe their symptoms. Anxiety and depression can also make people more generally introverted, withdrawn and isolated. In the case of autistic people this may be difficult to measure, as such individuals tend not to engage in much social activity outside the workplace anyway. All people with depression may have difficulty sharing their thoughts and feelings, but as people with autism can have difficulty labelling and sharing their feelings to start with, it can be especially hard to communicate symptoms or concerns. The combination of low self-esteem, a lack of confidence in themselves and the 'I really don't want to bother people' principle of what they might think must be a trivial issue to others (but not themselves) can only exacerbate the issue.

Treatments for severe depression can be psychological or medical, regardless of whether a person is autistic or not. The most important step to getting help is for the autistic person to tell someone they trust, such as a family member, a close friend, their GP or another professional. Some people need a referral to a specialist service, either because they would benefit from psychological therapy adapted for autistic people, or due to a more complex set of problems. Anxiety disorders, OCD and depression are just a few of the mental health problems people on the autism spectrum may experience.[29]

As autism, anxiety and depression are all closely linked, how much can psychotherapy or medication – or both – really help?

As with the matter of 'can autism be cured', there are two schools of thought – and perhaps one or more in between. Nick Dubin, who was diagnosed with Asperger syndrome at the age of twenty-seven and later wrote a book about his experiences, suggests that it is down to the individual. Only you can determine whether your anxiety has become such a problem that it has interfered with your ability to experience joy and happiness on a regular basis. An anxiety disorder, he writes, can often improve with insight, hard work, and even through certain prescribed medications, but sometimes these are not enough. The benefit of psychotherapy, he suggests, is that it can help to talk to somebody who can specifically help to address unique emotional issues, and a competent therapist can provide one with the individualised insight and feedback that cannot be acquired from any self-help books or the like.

With regard to medication, psychotherapeutic medications can sometimes be helpful in alleviating anxiety symptoms for those on the spectrum. Some drugs are noted for treating anxiety disorders, but they are not intended to do more than take the edge off anxiety, and they are not a cure. It all comes back to the question of what can and cannot be cured.[30]

Temple Grandin has written of the increasingly severe anxiety and panic attacks she experienced during her twenties. Hard exercise and physical work both helped her as a remedy, but she found that a low dose of antidepressants was the most effective of all, being essential to prevent side effects such as insomnia and agitation. Other people, she noted, found Prozac to be effective. Once more, it is less a case of cure and more one of helping to manage the condition more effectively. It is partly a matter of personal opinion, and partly deciding what works for the individual, and what does not.

Personally I tend to be a little sceptical about the use of medication in these instances. During a severe case of depression some years ago, I was given a prescription by my doctor. A few days ago my wife and a couple of members of the family undertook some online research into what I was taking, and we discovered that it could have some very unpleasant side effects. I stopped taking the pills that very day and the rest went straight in the bin. Moreover, after hearing from friends and others of the risks of getting addicted to prescription drugs and over-the-counter remedies, I tend to distance myself from such solutions as far as I possibly can. Having said that, I would not for a moment presume to sit in judgment about those for whom antidepressants really do work. To use a cliché, it is clearly not a case of 'one size fits all'.

Mental illness can be more common for people on the autism spectrum than in the general population, but the mental health of autistic people is often overlooked. Anxiety disorders are frequent among people on the autism spectrum, and it is estimated that about 40% have symptoms of at least one anxiety disorder at any one time, compared with up to 15% in the general population.

Anxiety can affect both the mind and the body, and produce a range of symptoms. The psychological and physical symptoms of anxiety are closely linked and can lead to a vicious cycle that can be difficult to break. The psychological symptoms of anxiety include easily losing patience, difficulty in concentrating, thinking persistently about the worst possible outcome to something, problems with sleeping properly, becoming preoccupied with or obsessive about one subject in particular, and above all depression. The physical symptoms include excessive thirst, stomach upsets, loose bowel movements, need to urinate more frequently than usual, periods of intensely pounding heart, headaches and muscular aching, dizzy spells, and pins and needles.

It is recommended that those who persistently or regularly experience any of these symptoms are recommended to seek medical advice, if only in order to rule out any other suspected medical conditions.

Anxiety is often only one step away from depression, or 'being in a dark place'. A combination of factors, leading to vulnerability to stress, can explain why anxiety disorders are so common in autistic people. Biological differences in brain structure and function, a history of social difficulties, leading to decreased self-esteem and a tendency to think of threats (sometimes imagined, or at the very least exaggerated) as greater than they are, and problems with finding flexible responses to apparent dark clouds on the horizon are all relevant factors.

People on the autism spectrum often have difficulty describing the symptoms they experience. This is the main reason why it is nearly always a task best left to a third party, such as a partner or parents if available, at the initial pre-diagnostic stage. A sudden change in behaviour might be a sign that they have developed an anxiety disorder, even or especially if there is no indication of any physical symptoms.

Most of the time we can learn to cope with difficult situations, whether we are autistic or not, often by 'riding the storm' or 'going with the flow' until matters improve of their own accord and we discover that we have not come to harm from the situation that worried us. However, people with anxiety disorder are more likely to try and escape from the situation, the result being a greater fear of the same and an even earlier escape the next time it occurs, as anxiety often takes root, builds on and reinforces itself. The solution is trying to break this cycle, and this is where cognitive (to do with thoughts) and – in particularly severe cases - behavioural psychological treatments can be as important in treatment as medication. These involve forming a working relationship with a therapist, building up any necessary skills, and working gently through a series of challenges involving exposure to an aspect of the situation one step at a time, that are anxiety-provoking but not intolerable. Together mind and body learn that the situation is not the horror it originally seemed to be, and this leads to a reduction in anxiety.

# OCD (obsessive compulsive disorder)

This anxiety disorder comprises obsessions and compulsions.

Obsessions are unwelcome thoughts, images, urges, worries or doubts that appear repeatedly in the mind and can result in anxiety or what is sometimes described as mental discomfort, a more mild term. They can interrupt your thoughts against your control and can be really frightening, graphic and disturbing. They may make you feel anxious, disgusted or 'mentally uncomfortable'. You might feel you cannot share them with others, or that there is something wrong with you that you have to hide. You do not choose to have obsessions - but you might feel upset that you are capable of having such thoughts. They can include fear of causing or failing to prevent harm, worrying you might have already harmed someone by not being careful enough, for example, that you have knocked someone over in your car, or worrying you are going to harm someone because you will lose control, perhaps by pushing someone in front of a train or stab them; intrusive thoughts, images and impulses of yourself doing something violent or abusive, leading you to worry that you are a dangerous person; religious or blasphemous thoughts that are against your normal religious beliefs; relationship intrusive thoughts that often appear as doubts about whether a relationship is right or whether you or your partner's feelings are strong enough, and which might lead you to end your relationship to get rid of the doubt and anxiety; fear of contamination by dirt or germs; mental contamination and uncomfortable feelings of 'internal uncleanliness'; fears and worries related to order or symmetry; fear that something bad will happen if everything is not clean, in perfect order or symmetrical.

Compulsions are repetitive activities that you do to alleviate the anxiety caused by the obsession. It could be something like repeatedly checking a door is locked, repeating a specific phrase in your head, or checking how your body feels. Compulsions are repetitive activities that you feel you have to do, the aim of a compulsion being to try and deal with the distress caused by obsessive thoughts. You might have to continue doing the compulsion until the anxiety goes away and things feel right again, while being aware that it makes no sense to carry out a compulsion, but you are afraid not to do it. Repeating compulsions is often time consuming and the relief they give does not last long. They can be physical actions, mental rituals, or involve a number, in that you might feel you have to complete a compulsion a specific number of times without being interrupted.[28]

It is thought to occur in about 2-3% of people who are not autistic, but much more commonly in those who are. Heredity or genes (DNA) and psychological predisposition can make people vulnerable to developing OCD, which can run in families. It can be distressing, exhausting and a severe hindrance in everyday life for sufferers and their families, but it is treatable. Sometimes wrongly mistaken for repetitive behaviour, it can be overlooked in people on the autism spectrum. Those who think they may have it should consult their GP, who will and can refer people for a specialised assessment to help work out what may be OCD and what may be autism instead. In recent years there has been increasing awareness of OCD, but it is still regarded as not acknowledged widely enough and therefore under-treated. If you are autistic and think that you may have OCD, it is best to get an assessment and treatment by a team that specialises in both autism and OCD.

The recommended treatments for OCD are Cognitive Behavioural Therapy (CBT) and medication. CBT gives you tools to help you change the way you think and act. As the most researched psychological treatment for OCD, there is now evidence that specialised CBT is effective for treating OCD and anxiety in people on the autism spectrum. Medication can be used either alone or in combination with CBT. The types of drugs usually prescribed for OCD are Selective Serotonin Reuptake Inhibitors, or SSRIs, and include Fluoxetine (Prozac) and Paroxetine (Seroxat). Some autistic people can be vulnerable to side-effects from medication and starting with a low dose is recommended. You and your doctor can increase this slowly over time if necessary, monitoring your symptoms with an OCD monitoring scale. Information about autism and

OCD (psychoeducation) and social skills work can also form part of a helpful package of individualised care for people on the autism spectrum and OCD.

# Case study 1: Becky Dowley

I was a little girl who used to watch the other children play in the school playground. I used to stand and hold the dinner ladies' hands and try to decipher how the children knew what to do. How did they know the rules? How did they have the confidence and know where they belonged? I had a group of boys I used to play with on the local estate but that did not require any negotiation or rules, we just to meet, run and hide and then go home again. The playground was a mass of screaming, running children who knew all the rules.

I was the little girl who cried every day after being left by my mum at primary school. I felt real, raw grief at having been removed from my nursery where I was safe and the climbing frame in the sunny garden was a haven. I missed my mum, my routine and the other children and couldn't navigate my way round this huge building with strangers everywhere. The teacher, an older woman, picked up a huge pile of books and hit me on the head with them to try to make me stop crying. I carried on crying every day, now with fear as well. I loved the school milk time and would sip the warm comforting nectar through the straw.

I was the little girl who drove my mum to distraction to the point where she took me to see a specialist who said I was 'gifted'. I was 3. I could read and write. I was hyperlexic and all the Peter and Jane books had been bought for me and read by the time I was 4.

I had two close friends as a slightly older girl, maybe 7, and these were Friend man 1 and Friend man 2. If this was today instead of 1976 the two men would be accused of all sorts but back in the day these were two completely innocent and quite beautiful friendships that evolved very naturally. Friend man 1 used to give me a large bag of small red apples every Saturday. He would wait outside his flat and pass them to me, smile his gummy smile and I would thank him and trot home with my prize. The apples were sweet and juicy and at a time when there was no spare money at home for sweets or treats, they were a prize indeed. Friend man 2 had snowy white hair and we used to sit in his garden and I would comment on his flowers whilst we drank tea from china tea cups and saucers. I can remember conversing with him about his lovely flower beds and sweet peas, I knew that it was important to praise him on their beauty as this would make him feel good. And they say us Autistics have no empathy.

I had what I now know is called Pica. I would eat play doh and the little beads from my small pink purse.

I was anxious and permanently crippling shy even with family. I felt on the periphery, on the side, not accepted, not worthy.

My mum was entrepreneurial in the feminist 1970s and 1980s. She was a single parent and she was bold and fierce. On the outside at least.

We moved to a guest house when I was 8 which was opposite the park and was a magnificent house with an even more magnificent garden. I spent hours in that garden on my own laying by the pond and watching the tadpoles or walking my doll round in her pram.

We moved to a café when I was 11 and there I met Friend man 3. He was sweet and old and used to drink tea and watch the cars go by where he would reminisce about his days as a mechanic. I know now he had Dementia.

I left home at 17 after a few tumultuous years arguing with my mum and moved in with a man who was nearly double my age and we spent all our time with people his age or older. We listened to music from the 1970s and despite not having any money or any prospects (I had dropped out of my A levels) we enjoyed simple pleasures.

I got a job as a nanny to two little boys and when the eldest was at school me and the baby had a wonderful four years of routine and solitude. Then he went to school and the bubble burst and I had to get a job in a care home. The routine kept me going.

We had a daughter who sadly died after being premature. Then we had a son. From day one this little baby would not settle, would not feed, would not be cuddled and was just not what the books had lead me to believe he would be like. From my nannying and experience I knew I could do this mothering thing well but he was just so squirmy and fidgety and unhappy. He couldn't feed from me, he didn't tolerate formula milk and ended up losing so much weight until he went onto soya milk. He had life threatening anaphylaxis and allergies and asthma and eczema. When we went shopping he would scream and kick and cry.

When he went to school he held the record for crying every day until Christmas. He went to school being able to write his name and the alphabet but he soon trailed behind his peers and the school would not listen to me when I said he was dyslexic. I seemed to not know this boy and yet intuitively understood him completely. I knew he wanted to just lay in his nappy and be free of clothing, I knew he needed routine, I knew he was just desperate to stay at home in the safety all day.

He loved dinosaurs and pokemon and bey blades. All the little boys did. Except with him he had to have the latest one then, not tomorrow or next week but then. And if he didn't get them he would be relentless until he got them. Still his letters were spelled backwards and his reading was non-existent, the school would not listen. We paid for a private test. He was dyslexic. No surprises. The school did not help. He would play with other children in his class when we met at the weekends, but only if he controlled the game and all the characters in it.

In amongst all this my life had moved on. I had met and married my husband and we had had a daughter. She was the complete opposite of my son and she just laid in my arms gazing at me and was cute and easy and sweet.

Time moved on, I went to University and worked and had my children and lived very happily with my husband. I became a teacher. The routine suited me.

Then one summer I had a new student coming to study on my programme and he had Asperger's syndrome. I decided to read up on it to ensure his success. As I read Tony Attwood's book I began to recognise my son. He was by now 16 and not very easy to live with. Sometimes slipping into an American accent when he was moody, easily overloaded, not having his food touching on his plate, argumentative and not liking being touched, I was reading his life in these pages. Crunch time came when he showed no empathy at all around my mother's cancer diagnosis and I spoke frankly to him about the fact that I thought he had Asperger's syndrome. I had written a list of all symptoms I thought he had. To my surprise he agreed to come to the doctors and she referred us to CAHMS (Child and Adolescent Mental Health Services). We were seen fairly quickly and the psychologist asked my son a few questions and then told him to pull his socks up. My son looked down and replied that his socks were pulled up and in that instant I realised that he was on the Autistic spectrum. Just like when an optical illusion snaps into focus, my perspective on life changed irreversibly. About a year later he got his diagnosis and I was relieved and grieved and set about to educate myself.

As with so many women I read everything I could get my hands on to empower both him and me. I soaked information up and got lots of books out of the library. One day sitting in bed reading and note taking I read about a little girl who would not play in the playground and who had older people as friends. I read about not liking the hoover noise or the hand drier noise. I read about being nervous when travelling on the train. I thought about how I felt like an outsider all the time, like I was trying to fit in but not quite making it. How I only have a couple of friends and they are spread all around the country. How at my dyslexia test at work the previous year the assessor had said to me 'You're a bit odd really aren't you?' and written on the report that in some of the areas tested I was off the scale because I had been so bright, and in other tests I was off the scale because I read out loud so slowly that there wasn't a measure for it.

After a while I started to notice things about myself. Things like how if I was due to meet someone at 11 a.m., then 11 a.m. was when they should arrive. Not two minutes past or two minutes to. I noticed that I did a lot of stimming. I noticed that my aversion to eye contact was actually quite noticeable. How I had been so wrapped up in ensuring that my son's food didn't touch on the plate that I hadn't noticed that if a sandwich had a slight bit of soggy bread I couldn't even look at it let alone eat it. The hoover scares me, hand driers scare me.

I went to the same GP I had gone to with my son with my list in my hand. She referred me and a year later my trips down to St Austell started. I had to go on the train on my own which was a major ordeal. I wore the same jean skirt and top for all visits. I had the same taxi driver when I got off the train and sat in the same seat at the station cafe to have a cup of tea and a Twix before my appointment. Safety in routine.

And then came the day of my diagnosis, a lovely hot sunny day in late July. I was nervous because I thought that the psychologist was going to say that I was just shy and had a few quirks. However in actual fact she produced a report which said that I fulfilled every area of diagnosis fully and that she rarely saw someone with so many characteristics. I cried. She asked why I cried. I said I didn't know but I thought it might be relief.

On the way home I read the report that she had prepared. It was very detailed and reflected everything I had told her and all the tests that she had carried out.

Here was I, a wife, a mother, a foster mother, a teacher, a colleague, a friend, an aunt, a sister, a mentor, a godmother and now an Autistic.

I was shell-shocked. Yet I was liberated, freed, released, delighted, vindicated, recognised, validated and felt I had been seen for the first time as me.

Interestingly in the report there was a large section on my mum with whom I had had a difficult relationship and who had died the previous year. With whom everyone had had a difficult relationship. My psychologist had, from my accounts, tentatively written that with some of mum's odd little ways, she could well have been on the spectrum. My mum suddenly became someone I could understand. The woman who flinched if you hugged her. Who screamed when the doorbell rang. Who had no friends come to her funeral.

I told people of my diagnosis very slowly. Some people said that they already knew I was Autistic. Some people refuted it. Some people said that we are all a bit Autistic (we are not). Now all my colleagues know, my friends know, my husband and children know, the difference is now I don't really mind who knows because it is a part of me as my eye colour or my shoe size.

Now, four summers on I am a changed person. I am accepting of who I am. I am still that little girl who stood in the playground holding the dinner ladies hand but now I know why. I still get awkward in a one to one conversation unless I know you very well. I will still not share my pens with you. I will not eat a pre-prepared sandwich. I had trouble driving somewhere that I don't know. I don't like talking on the phone even to family. I will dry my hands on tissue rather than use the hand drier. But I know why and so I push my limits every day.

I am just completing a Masters in Autism and next year I hope to start a Doctorate. I am the author of two published articles, a blog and have been asked to speak at a conference in November.

Autism has been the most difficult and the most liberating aspect of my life. No one see's the struggles I go through every day, but I know they are there and despite it being exhausting I push myself every day to be the best I can be.

# Case study 2: Abi G on her father

My father is 76 years old. In his youth as a beatnik, he was living rough for a while, drinking and taking drugs. When found living in a church he was taken to task by Her Majesty's Prisons. My grandad was disgusted and kept him out of jail on the promise of a good hiding and clean living, ha!

He worked on the roads as a joiner for a few years after travelling for a long time, and ended up in Plymouth with a small family. After searching for further work he discovered his passion for teaching. He never got a job as a geology or geography teacher, but ended up as a poetry fanatic teaching English in a secondary modern school. It was not quite what he expected.

Over the years us kids have been privy to his strange ways. Signing pencils out officially from his pencil box, and decimalisation for categorising our own kids' books - my dad's a library fanatic. Days out in book shops or Dartmoor ONLY buying three copies of one book; one for bookcase which can't be moved, touched or otherwise, one for cutting up and rewriting as the grammar is tripe, and last one for reading for pleasure although he never read a novel in his life, all science and info rather than romance and true life. I found out recently that he only has ever cleaned his teeth once a day, finding it absolutely amazing that twice was the norm - what did my mum ever teach him, I wonder?

He has worn the same hi-tech trainers for over 30 years and never attended a gym. When hi-techs were no longer available, he moved on to walking trainers for his travels, same colour, shape, and any changes to the lace design drive him mad. He used to camp a lot, and everything he took in his backpack was weighed for tightness and sawn to its smallest length. He has over twenty-five rucksacks and several dozen sleeping bags that he won't let me give to the homeless in case he needs them.

He smokes nineteen fags a day, one left in the packet for the morning, same every day since he was fifteen years old. Should this system go astray, he has been known to be unable to sleep, and back in the 1970s he would walk across Plymouth to find the only petrol station to be open to buy more. He never diverts from the brand, then suddenly like most things he changes and will never return to the old brands for no apparent reason.

More recently it took us two years to get him to buy new double-glazed windows even when his old Victorian windows were cracked and missing. As he was working on one of his many projects, we rag him about the shares he should have in the shop Staples. He has over 500 files, once golden in colour. A change from Staples meant an entire move now to sage, all perfectly good golden ones swapped and wrapped up and God help the person who makes any design changes. A sage satin finish does not match a sage shiny one - you catch my drift.

He always shops at ASDA and buys chops, carrots, mince, potatoes and onions in huge bags that go mouldy, and meat that sits in the fridge bloody for weeks. He has a huge filing system for recorded programmes which he never watches, but goes mad if anyone touches them or the TV set up specifically to record stationed where else but in the spare room, he has another TV for watching and a third for watching old videos. Emotionally he understands little but he can often be amusing. His sense of smell is odd.

I'm running out of time - excuse the lengthy witterings – oh, he also has OCD. The GP told him about eighteen months ago, when he finally told him I thought he had autism and I was probably talking rubbish, he was little surprised. His GP agreed. He couldn't get his head around that, and he still declines the diagnosis of autism. His projects are his life and they take over anything including family at times always.

I do love his oddness though.

# Acknowledgements

My thanks are due to several people.

Kerry Kellaway, alongside whom I worked for two and a half years, was not only very supportive throughout but also encouraged me when I told her I was planning to write this book, agreeing wholeheartedly that there was a need for such a title, and agreed to add some words on her experiences of me as an autistic colleague.

Becky Dowley and Abi G, who taught at the organisation where I was working, have had personal or close family experience of autism and were kind enough to contribute case histories.

Rebecca Finch allowed me to read her university dissertation on the subject and quote some of her thoughts.

My friends Ian Herne and Nikki Geary, one from my student days and the other also a former colleague at work, were very helpful with suggestions while I was putting it all together.

My greatest debut goes to my wife, who put her finger on the problem in the first place.

# Reference Notes

All websites accessed between June 2017 and
May 2018

1 Coughlan, Sean, 'Why shouldn't I be autistic
and a student?' BBC News online, 27 April 2018;
http://www.bbc.co.uk/news/education-43912447

2 Wood, Ruth, 'Autism: It provides an
explanation for feeling 'different'', *Daily
Telegraph*, 29 June 2015

3 Snedden, Robert, *Explaining Autism* (Franklin
Watts, 2008)

4 Canavan, Cary, *Supporting pupils on the autism
spectrum in secondary schools* (Routledge, 2015)

5 Dubin, Nick, *Asperger syndrome and anxiety*
(Jessica Kingsley Publishers, 2009)

6 The Exclusive Inclusive Employment Hub blog
https://incluzy.com/autism/the-difference-
between-autism-and-aspergers/

7 Watkins, Lynne, *My A to Z of Living with
Asperger's Syndrome and Autism* (lulu.com,
2014)

8 'Information for people who have been diagnosed with an Autism Spectrum Condition' (Devon Autism & ADHD Service, c.2012)

9 Paxton, Katherine, and Estay, Irene A., *Counselling People on the Autism Spectrum: A Practical Manual* (Jessica Kingsley Publishers, 2007)

10 Finch, Rebecca, *A Lived Experience of Autism Spectrum Disorder* (Dissertation, University of Teesside, 2015)

11 Temple Grandin, FAQ, accessed July 2017 http://www.templegrandin.com/faq.html

12 Attwood, Tony, *The Complete Guide to Asperger's Syndrome* (Jessica Kingsley Publishers, 2007)

13 Drew, Gillan, *An Adult With An Autism Diagnosis: A Guide for the Newly Diagnosed* (Jessica Kingsley Publishers, 2017)

14 Peel, John, and Ravenscroft, Sheila, *Margrave of the Marshes* (Bantam Press, 2005)

15 Brown, Julie, *Writers on the Spectrum: How Autism and Asperger Syndrome Have Influenced Literary Writing* (Jessica Kingsley Publishers, 2010)

16 Lockyer, Daphne, 'Award-winning actor Paddy Considine talks for the first time about being diagnosed with Asperger's – at the age of 36.' *Daily Telegraph*, 10 April 2011

17 Wintle, Angela, 'Gary Numan: My family values.' *Guardian*, 5 May 2012; https://autism-connect.org.uk/users/blogDetail/5643751d88916

18 National Autism website http://www.autism.org.uk/chrispackham

19 Deveney, Catherine, 'Susan Boyle: my relief at discovering that I have Asperger's', *Guardian*, 8 December 2013

20 Eliot, Marc, *Paul Simon: A life* (John Wiley, 2010)

21 Older people with autism in Scotland 'invisible' 02/10/2013 https://www.connecttosupport.org/s4s/NewsArticleCmsContext/View/300e4727-751e-425a-8c56-a24900b16109?Page=23

22 Sinclair, Jim, 'Don't mourn for us', Autism Network International newsletter, *Our Voice*, Vol 1, No 3, 1993.

23 *Research Autism website* http://researchautism.net/autism/adults-on-the-autism-spectrum/interventions-for-adults-on-the-autism-spectrum

24 Hendrickx, Sarah, & Tinsley, Matthew, *Asperger Syndrome and Alcohol: Drinking to Cope?* (Jessica Kingsley, 2008); Autism and alcohol, 2016, Network Autism website, http://network.autism.org.uk/good-practice/case-studies/autism-and-alcohol

25 BBC Radio 4 Woman's Hour, 4 January 2017

26 Mills, Richard, Reflections on stress and autism,
http://network.autism.org.uk/good-practice/evidence-base/reflections-stress-and-autism

27 Obsessive compulsive disorder, MIND website
https://www.mind.org.uk/information-support/types-of-mental-health-problems/obsessive-compulsive-disorder-ocd/symptoms-of-ocd/#obsessions

28 Sarris, Marina, *Diagnosing Depression In Autism* (2016), Interactive Autism Network
https://iancommunity.org/diagnosing-depression-autism

29 NHS choices website,
http:///www.nhs.uk/Conditions/Anxiety/Pages/Symptoms.aspx

30 Galanopoulos, Dr Anastasios, Robertson, Dr Dene, Spain, Debbie and Murphy, Dr Clodagh. Mental Health supplement, *Your Autism Magazine*, Vol 8 (4), Winter 2014
http://www.autism.org.uk/about/health/mental health.aspx